Hypertrophic Cardiomyopathy

For patients, their families and
interested physicians

Hypertrophic Cardiomyopathy

FOR PATIENTS, THEIR FAMILIES AND INTERESTED PHYSICIANS

Second Edition

By
Barry J. Maron, MD
Director
The Hypertrophic Cardiomyopathy Center
Minneapolis Heart Institute Foundation
Minneapolis, MN, USA

Lisa Salberg
President
Hypertrophic Cardiomyopathy Association
Hibernia, NJ, USA

The second edition of this popular book is for the use and benefit of patients afflicted with hypertrophic cardiomyopathy, their families, and treating physicians, and with a commitment to the dissemination of information regarding this complex and often misunderstood disease.

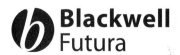

© 2001 Futura Media Services, Inc, New York
© 2006 Barry J. Maron and Lisa Salberg
Published by Blackwell Publishing
Blackwell Futura is an imprint of Blackwell Publishing

Blackwell Publishing, Inc., 350 Main Street, Malden, Massachusetts 02148-5020, USA
Blackwell Publishing Ltd, 9600 Garsington Road, Oxford OX4 2DQ, UK
Blackwell Science Asia Pty Ltd, 550 Swanston Street, Carlton, Victoria 3053, Australia

First published 2001
Second edition 2006

3   2008

Library of Congress Cataloging-in-Publication Data

Maron, Barry J. (Barry Joel), 1941-
   Hypertrophic cardiomyopathy : for patients, their families, and interested physicians /
by Barry J. Maron and Lisa Salberg.—2nd ed.
      p. cm.
   "The second edition of this popular book is for the use and benefit of patients
afflicted with hypertrophic cardiomyopathy, their families and treating physicians, and
with a commitment to the dissemination of information regarding this uncommon,
complex and often misunderstood disease."
   Includes bibliographical references.
   ISBN : 978-1-4051-4710-1
1. Heart—Hypertrophy. I. Salberg, Lisa. II. Title.

RC685.H9M27 2006
616.1'24—dc22

                                                                    2006018504

ISBN: 978-1-4051-4710-1

A catalogue record for this title is available from the British Library

Acquisitions: Gina Almond
Development: Beckie Brand
Set in 10/13 Palatino by Charon Tec Ltd, Chennai, India
Printed and bound by Sheridan Books, Inc. in Ann Arbor, Michagan

For further information on Blackwell Publishing, visit our website:
www.blackwellcardiology.com

Contents

Acknowledgments

I wish to acknowledge the constant and ongoing support, which made this book (and all the HCM papers) possible, for more than 35 years – from my wife Donna and our two boys, Dr. Marty Maron and Dr. Bradley Maron (who are physicians), as well as our daughter-in-law, Dr. Jill Maron. I also wish to acknowledge our two grandchildren Alexis (age 2 years) and Jack Maron (age 6 months), who have not yet applied to medical school.

Barry J. Maron MD
Minneapolis, MN

Dedication

This book is dedicated to my entire family for their continued support, and specifically to my husband, Adam, and my daughter, Becca. I love you both "all the way to the moon and back." This book is also dedicated to the memory of those lost to HCM, including my sister, Lori, and dear friend, Carolyn Biro, and in honor of the thousands of those LIVING with HCM every day.

Thank you to Dr. Barry J. Maron and all the HCMA Medical Advisors and Board of Directors for their friendship, support, and tireless efforts on behalf of HCM patients around the world. Special thanks to Kelly DeRosa for all of her efforts.

Lisa Salberg
Rockaway Township, NJ

Foreword

Almost a half century ago, while I was training in cardiology at the National Institutes of Health (NIH), my colleagues and I encountered two young men with obstruction to the outflow of blood from the heart's main pumping chamber, the left ventricle. The condition was quite mysterious since the cause of the obstruction was not clear and the available medical literature was unhelpful. With the passage of time, our group at the NIH and other cardiologists and cardiovascular surgeons around the world recognized an increasing number of such patients and learned that this condition, now called hypertrophic cardiomyopathy (HCM), could present in a wide variety of ways. However, it was thought at first that obstruction was a *sine qua non* of HCM and that the prognosis was guarded.

As a result of extensive and carefully conducted research by many talented scientists and clinicians, the veil surrounding this condition has been lifted and we now know that rather than a medical curiosity, HCM is, in fact, the most common genetic cardiac disease. It occurs in approximately 1 in every 500 persons, more than half a million patients in the United States alone. The abnormal genes responsible in the majority of patients with HCM have been discovered and can be tested for. Screening and diagnosis can be accomplished readily with an ultrasound examination. Perhaps most importantly, it has been established that most patients can lead normal or near normal lives. Management can be "tailored" to individual patients; many require nothing more than lifestyle modification and careful follow up examinations. In other patients symptoms can be managed with commonly used drugs, such as the familiar beta blockers. Serious disturbances of cardiac rhythm can often be aborted with implanted defibrillators. An operation, surgical myomectomy, pioneered at the NIH more than 40 years ago, is reserved for patients with severe symptomatic obstruction and has improved steadily over the years. The risk of the procedure is now very low when it is carried out in experienced institutions.

This exceptionally well written "short book" on HCM describes the nature of the disease, the implications of genetic transmission, as well as the methods of screening, diagnosis and estimating prognosis. All forms of treatment, their indications and risks are discussed. Importantly, this book provides useful recommendations on lifestyle, sports and pregnancy.

The authors bring their extensive experience to this book. Dr. Maron has devoted his professional life to the study of and research into HCM and he shares his immense knowledge with the reader. Ms. Salberg, a patient with HCM, who is the founder and President of the HCM Association, provides the critically important perspectives of patients and their families. This lucid and understandable book will be of enormous value to patients with HCM, their families and caregivers, including physicians. Dr. Maron and Ms. Salberg deserve profound thanks for devoting their talents and efforts to this important project.

Eugene Braunwald, MD
Brigham and Women's Hospital
Harvard Medical School
Boston, Massachusetts.

Introduction

The second edition of this handbook is designed (as was the initial version) for those interested in understanding the cardiac condition, hypertrophic cardiomyopathy (or HCM). The manuscript was created through the collaboration of expert physicians, other medical personnel including nurses, and patients with the disease, and seeks to address the major questions and concerns about HCM. We also believe this book will be useful to physicians (including cardiologists) in developing an understanding of HCM. While the language of the text was designed largely with non-medically oriented individuals in mind (medical terminology and jargon are kept to a minimum and very basic anatomy and physiology is discussed), this editorial strategy should not discourage medical personnel at any level from using and benefiting from the information contained herein.

Therefore, this book is not intended to be an elementary document describing a complex condition, but rather a scientific treatise written and organized in such a way to be appropriate and accessible to as wide an audience as possible, including patients without medical or scientific background. Every effort has been made in this second edition to take into account the rapid changes and enhanced knowledge regarding HCM which has evolved over the past 5 years. Therefore, the clinical concepts presented here concerning HCM can be regarded as relevant, important, and up to date. Patients are cautioned that this book is an effort to describe the entire disease spectrum of HCM in a comprehensive fashion and therefore much of the information contained herein may not directly or explicitly pertain to some patients.

What is hypertrophic cardiomyopathy (HCM)?

Cardiomyopathy is a general term describing any condition in which the heart muscle is structurally and functionally abnormal (the heart itself is, of course, a specialized type of muscle). While there are many types of cardiomyopathy, many of which are genetic and familial, we are concerned here with only *hypertrophic cardiomyopathy (HCM)*.

HCM is a genetic disease affecting the heart muscle. The most consistent feature of HCM is excessive thickening of that portion of the heart muscle known as the left ventricle (heart muscle thickening = *hypertrophy*; diseased heart muscle = *cardiomyopathy*). In quantitative terms, hypertrophy is usually defined as a wall thickness of 15 mm or more when measured by ultrasound (echocardiogram). The consequences of HCM to patients are related, in part or solely, to the abnormally thickened left ventricular heart muscle which in turn is a consequence of the basic genetic defect. Hypertrophy may be widespread throughout the left ventricle, but may also be more limited in distribution, and there is no single pattern of muscle thickening which is "typical" of HCM. The region of the left ventricle which is usually the site of the most prominent thickening is the ventricular septum; that is, that portion of muscle which separates the left and right ventricular cavities.

The heart (specifically the left ventricle) may also thicken in other individuals who do not have HCM, either as a result of high blood pressure, obstructive heart valve disease, or even prolonged and intense athletic training in certain sports. The type of hypertrophy associated with high blood pressure is often referred to as secondary (i.e., a consequence of the increased blood pressure). In HCM, however, the muscular thickening of the heart wall is *primary* – that is, due to a genetic defect and not a reaction to other factors.

In addition, when the heart muscle of HCM is viewed under a light microscope, it usually shows several particular abnormalities, the most prominent of which is called *myocardial cell (myocyte) disarray or disorganization* (Figure 1), in which normal parallel alignment of heart muscle cells has been lost and many of the muscle cells are arranged in a characteristically chaotic and disorganized pattern. It is likely that this cell disarray interferes with normal electrical transmission of impulses and predisposes some patients to irregularities of heart rhythm, as well as

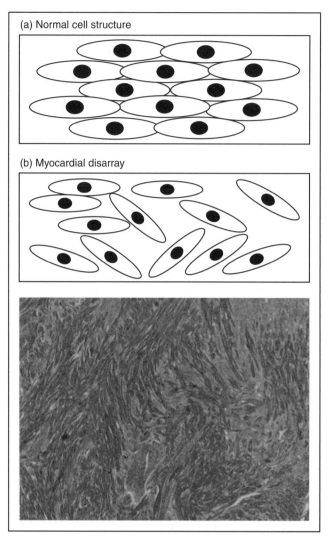

Figure 1 *The cell structure and architecture of the HCM heart.* Diagrams contrast the regular and parallel alignment of muscle cells in the normal heart (a) with the irregular, disorganized alignment of cells ("myocardial disarray") found in some areas of the HCM heart (b). At the bottom is a micrograph of an actual area of an HCM heart (from a histologic section) showing the disorganized and chaotic arrangement of cardiac muscle cells (myocytes).

altering the heart contraction. In addition, there are often scars (comprised of collagen; i.e., fibrosis of various size and extent within the wall of the left ventricle), which probably result from inadequate blood supply to the heart muscle.

Historical perspective and names

The first modern description of HCM was in 1958 by a British pathologist, Dr. Donald Teare, who likened the disease to a tumor of the heart. However, there is some evidence that HCM was initially recognized in the mid-1850s by German and French investigators. Nevertheless, over these many years the condition has been known by a vast number of names. Indeed, this issue of nomenclature *is* often confusing to patients and even some physicians (Figure 2).

Remarkably, HCM has been given over 75 separate names or designations by individual clinicians and scientists over the last almost 50 years (Figure 2). Literally, no other disease can make that claim. Why has this occurred? The principal reason for the proliferation of names undoubtedly has been the heterogeneity and diversity with which HCM is expressed, a major point in ultimately understanding this disease. Also, since very few cardiologists have treated large numbers of patients with HCM, they often came to regard the overall disease based solely on their personal (and sometimes limited) experiences.

Many of the alternate names for HCM emphasize obstruction to left ventricular outflow, which is a highly visible feature of the disease. Obstruction is probably present under resting conditions in just 25% of all patients; however, about 70% of all HCM patients have the capacity for obstruction, either at rest or (if not present at rest) when provoked by physiologic exercise. Therefore, names for this disease have included IHSS (or idiopathic hypertrophic subaortic *stenosis*) which was the first popular term used in the United States ("stenosis" means obstruction). The same can be said for HOCM (hypertrophic obstructive cardiomyopathy) which is still widely used in the United Kingdom. Indeed, you may well hear your disease referred to by more than the designation … HCM.

Presently, virtually all HCM experts and other cardiovascular specialists now regard *hypertrophic cardiomyopathy* (or *HCM*) as the best single name for the broad disease spectrum. This term emphasizes the *hypertrophy* which is the diagnostic marker in most patients and the fact that this disease is a *cardiomyopathy* – or heart muscle disorder – and without mentioning obstruction (which is *not* present in each patient). Therefore, the terms "HCM *with* obstruction" or "HCM *without* obstruction" are preferred.

Terms used to describe hypertrophic cardiomyopathy

Acquired aortic subvalvular stenosis
Apical asymmetric septal hypertrophy
Apical hypertrophic cardiomyopathy
Apical hypertrophic nonobstructive cardiomyopathy
Apical hypertrophy
Asymmetric left ventricular hypertrophy
Asymmetric septal hypertrophy
Asymmetrical apical hypertrophy
Asymmetrical hypertrophic cardiomyopathy
Asymmetrical hypertrophy of the heart
Asymmetrical septal hypertrophy (ASH)
Brock's disease
Diffuse muscular subaortic stenosis
Diffuse subvalvular aortic stenosis
Dynamic hypertrophic subaortic stenosis
Dynamic muscular subaortic stenosis
Familial hypertrophic subaortic stenosis
Familial hypertrophic cardiomyopathy
Familial muscular subaortic stenosis
Familial myocardial disease
Functional aortic stenosis
Functional aortic subvalvular stenosis
Functional hypertrophic subaortic stenosis
Functional obstructive cardiomyopathy
Functional obstruction of the left ventricle
Functional obstructive subvalvular aortic stenosis
Functional subaortic stenosis
Hereditary cardiovascular dysplasia

Hypertrophic apical cardiomyopathy
HYPERTROPHIC CARDIOMYOPATHY (HCM)
Hypertrophic constrictive cardiomyopathy
Hypertrophic disease
Hypertrophic hyperkinetic cardiomyopathy
Hypertrophic infundibular aortic stenosis
Hypertrophic nonobstructive apical cardiomyopathy
Hypertrophic nonobstructive cardiomyopathy
Hypertrophic nonobstructive cardiomyopathy
Hypertrophic obstructive cardiomyopathy with giant negative T-waves
Hypertrophic obstructive cardiomyopathy
Hypertrophic obstructive cardiomyopathy of the left ventricle
Hypertrophic restrictive cardiomyopathy
Hypertrophic stenosing cardiomyopathy
Hypertrophic subaortic stenosis
Idiopathic hypertrophic cardiomyopathy
Idiopathic hypertrophic obstructive cardiomyopathy
Idiopathic hypertrophic subaortic stenosis (IHSS)
Idiopathic hypertrophic subvalvular stenosis
Idiopathic muscular hypertrophic subaortic stenosis
Idiopathic muscular stenosis of the left ventricle
Idiopathic myocardial hypertrophy
Idiopathic stenosis of the flushing chamber of the left ventricle
Idiopathic ventricular septal hypertrophy
Irregular hypertrophic cardiomyopathy
Left ventricular muscular stenosis

Low subvalvular aortic stenosis
Mid-ventricular hypertrophic cardiomyopathy
Mid-ventricular hypertrophic obstructive cardiomyopathy
Mid-ventricular obstruction
Muscular aortic stenosis
Muscular hypertrophic stenosis of the left ventricle
Muscular stenosis of the left ventricle
Muscular subaortic stenosis
Muscular subvalvular aortic stenosis
Non-dilated cardiomyopathy
Nonobstructive hypertrophic cardiomyopathy
Obstructive cardiomyopathy
Obstructive hypertrophic aortic stenosis
Obstructive hypertrophic cardiomyopathy
Obstructive hypertrophic myocardiopathy
Obstructive myocardiopathy
Pseudoaortic stenosis
Stenosing hypertrophy of the left ventricle
Stenosis of the ejection chamber of the left ventricle
Subaortic hypertrophic obstructive cardiomyopathy
Subaortic hypertrophic stenosis
Subaortic idiopathic stenosis
Subaortic muscular stenosis
Subvalvular aortic stenosis
Subvalvular aortic stenosis of the muscular type
Teare's disease
Typical hypertrophic obstructive cardiomyopathy

Figure 2 HCM has acquired many names (about 75) in four decades which reflects the diversity with which the disease is expressed. Hypertrophic cardiomyopathy is the preferred name at this time.

How common is HCM?

HCM has the reputation as a rare disease. However, a number of recent population studies from the United States and elsewhere show that HCM is a more common disease than previously regarded. It is now estimated that about 1 in 500 individuals within the general population have this disease. HCM is truly a global disease and these prevalence figures come from populations as diverse as the United States, Japan, and China (Figure 3). These figures relate to adults in whom the disease is recognized by echocardiography (i.e., by visualizing the thickening of the left ventricular wall). However, many other children and adults could carry a mutant gene for HCM and not be easily detectable by echocardiography or not come to clinical recognition for a variety of reasons (including absence of a heart murmur and obstruction), and therefore be completely unaware of their diagnosis. Indeed, the 1 in 500 prevalence figure is likely to be an *underestimation* given the large number of genetically affected individuals in HCM families with little or no overt clinical evidence of the disease.

Indeed, the currently recognized HCM patient population has been likened to the "tip of the iceberg" with most affected patients undiagnosed and unknown "below the surface" (Figure 4). This helps explain why HCM seems so uncommon in cardiology practice (i.e., why cardiologists so often

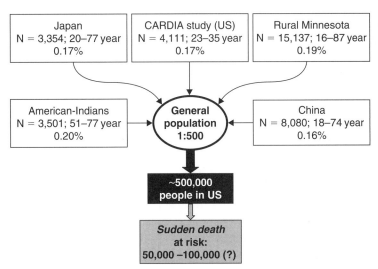

Figure 3 The stated prevalence of 1:500 for HCM is based on actual population data in several cohorts from different parts of the world.

HCM: the tip of the iceberg

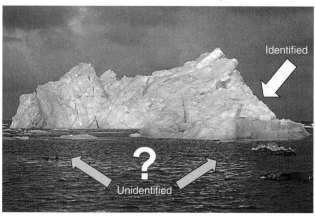

Figure 4 The HCM patients who are currently recognized clinically represent the "tip of the iceberg" – that is, a minority of the overall HCM population. Therefore, most patients remain undiagnosed.

tell HCM patients they only occasionally see this condition), but in fact is the most common genetic cardiac disease. This large number of names used to describe HCM may be one factor responsible for the perceived low visibility of HCM in the public sector relative to other less common diseases. In fact, HCM is much more common (and has a major impact on the public health) than "better known" non-cardiac conditions such as cystic fibrosis, multiple sclerosis, muscular dystrophy, and amyotrophic lateral sclerosis (ALS; Lou Gehrig disease) or cardiovascular diseases such as Marfans syndrome (Figure 5). These other conditions in most cases are truly rare, occurring in only 1:10,000 or less, while HCM is the most common genetic heart disease and cause of sudden death in the young – occurring in 1:500 people (Figure 5).

HCM appears to occur throughout the world with most of the scientific interest and reports from North America (United States and Canada), the Far East (Japan, China, Australia), and Europe (United Kingdom, Italy, France, Germany, Switzerland), although there is increasing attention to HCM in Brazil, Argentina, Chile, Israel, and New Zealand. HCM appears to be remarkably similar with regard to clinical presentation, heart structure and prognosis in patients from these diverse areas of the world. One relatively minor exception is the apical form of HCM (with wall thickening localized to the tip [apex] of the left ventricle) which is always without obstruction and seems to be more common in Japan – but is not at all limited to Asians – a distinction which could reflect unique racial, ethnic, and/or environmental

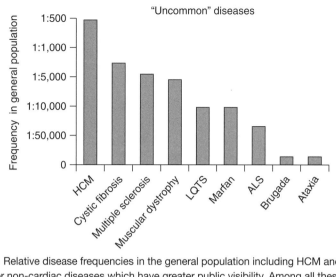

Figure 5 Relative disease frequencies in the general population including HCM and other cardiac or non-cardiac diseases which have greater public visibility. Among all these diseases, HCM is distinctly more common. ALS: amyotrophic lateral sclerosis; LQTS: long QT syndrome.

factors. This structural form is not a separate disease entity and occurs in 3% of U.S. (non-Asian) patients.

What is the cause of HCM?

It is important to emphasize that HCM is usually a familial condition and represents a genetically transmitted disease. The pattern of inheritance for HCM is known as ***autosomal dominant***, which means that the disease (and the mutant gene) appears in about 50% of the members in each consecutive generation. Therefore, the likelihood of an affected parent transmitting the abnormal gene to their child is statistically about one in two (Figure 6). However, autosomal dominant inheritance does not necessarily mean that if there are 4 offsprings, 2 must be affected – only that this is the statistical probability. In reality, it could be 0 of 4 or even 4 of 4 offspring who will carry the mutant gene. In addition, some individuals with this disease appear to be "sporadic" cases – that is, there are no other relatives in the family known to have clinical evidence of HCM, or one of the known genetic markers. There is always the possibility of a *de novo* (new) mutation – that is, the first member of the family with the mutant gene and disease.

Generations

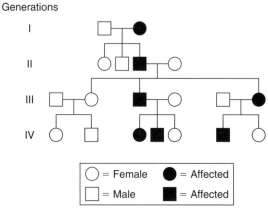

Figure 6 *Family tree*. Shown here are four generations of a family affected by HCM. There is typical *autosomal dominant inheritance* in which the condition is transmitted from one generation to another. In each generation every offspring of an affected person has a 50% chance of inheriting the gene and disease.

Genetic "skipping" of a generation is rare but can appear to occur when an individual who is a gene carrier does not have evidence of HCM on the echocardiogram. In such a circumstance, the defective gene does not actually "skip" a generation – but in reality the HCM gene in that individual simply does not express itself fully so that evidence of the disease can be visualized with the echocardiogram (known as "incomplete penetrance").

At present, a multitude of about 400 mutations in 11 genes, which are necessary for the development and contraction of heart muscle cells (in units called **sarcomeres**), have been mapped to their respective chromosomes and isolated from members of families with HCM (some of these mutations also exist in skeletal muscle, as well as heart muscle). The 11 genes presently regarded as causing HCM are known in scientific terms as: (1) beta-myosin heavy chain; (2) myosin-binding protein C; (3) troponin-T; (4) troponin-I; (5) alpha-tropomyosin; (6 and 7) essential and regulatory myosin light chains; (8) actin; (9) alpha-myosin heavy chain; (10) titin; and (11) muscle LIM protein. In most patients, HCM is caused by the initial three genes on this list while the other eight genes each account for only a small fraction of the patients. Indeed, this is one of the reasons HCM is widely regarded as a diverse and heterogeneous disease. Additional genes and mutations responsible for HCM will undoubtedly be identified in the future since the known mutant genes account for only about 50% of the overall patient population.

A *mutation* is a defect in the DNA code, the protein structure of the gene. These DNA abnormalities may take many forms, but some can be likened to a "spelling error" in the genetic code of DNA such as displacement in the order or sequence of just one of the many amino acids (the individual "building blocks" of the gene protein). Indeed, it is striking and perhaps surprising that such seemingly minor-appearing abnormalities in the gene sequence can make such a profound difference in the structure of the heart, as occurs in HCM.

Patients often inquire about the cause of their mutation, particularly if the gene abnormality has apparently appeared for the first time in a family (as a *de novo* mutation). This consideration usually arises when a newly diagnosed child has both parents with normal echocardiograms and no evidence of HCM. Keep in mind that the genetic predisposition to HCM (i.e., the mutant gene) does not always trace back many generations in the same family but may occur spontaneously and for the first time in a member of the most recent generation. At present, the environmental factors that may trigger HCM mutations are unknown.

The discovery of the gene defects responsible for HCM is a major step toward understanding in precise terms the basic cause of HCM. In addition, laboratory DNA diagnosis from a blood test is now available for the first time commercially. This availability may prove to be particularly useful in identifying HCM in young children and adolescents, in patients with hypertension, or in clinical situations where the HCM diagnosis is ambiguous – such as athletes in whom it is difficult to distinguish HCM from the effects of chronic exercise and training on the heart (i.e., "athlete's heart").

This type of genetic testing has also been utilized selectively by families with a known HCM mutation to determine if their children or other relatives have the same genetic marker. This knowledge will allow for careful follow-up for those with a known genetic mutation or freedom from the need for annual cardiac evaluation in those relatives without a mutation. Certainly, the knowledge of a "mutation" may be highly emotional, debilitating, and in some ways even worse than an actual diagnosis for a particular patient. Genetic counseling is highly recommended for family members undergoing genetic screening to prepare them for the results and help interpret the findings.

Ongoing and future investigations will focus on the identification of new genes that cause HCM and ultimately on understanding how these genetic abnormalities operate in formulating HCM. While the effort to distinguish "good" and "bad" HCM genes continues (with the eventual goal of isolating those patients who are at high risk for sudden death or disease progression), at present this information is incomplete and it is not possible to make routine assessments of prognosis from this test.

Some molecular biologists focused on HCM are of the view that knowledge of the basic genetic defect in individual families will ultimately unlock many of the important secrets of this disease and permit more targeted, definitive, and earlier therapeutic interventions. However, such a level of complete understanding is many years (and perhaps many decades) off, and until that time cardiologists must advise and treat patients with the available practical, clinical strategies – some of which are, in fact, powerful and efficacious.

At the time of publication of this book the Genetic Information Non-discrimination Act (S. 306, H.R. 1227) is pending in the U.S. Congress. The Act will prohibit discrimination on the basis of genetic information with respect to health insurance and employment. It was introduced to establish basic legal protections that will enable and encourage individuals to take advantage of genetic screening, counseling, testing, and new therapies that will result from the scientific advances in the field of genetics. It would also prevent health insurers from denying coverage or adjusting premiums based on an individual's predisposition to a genetic condition, and prohibit employers from discriminating on the basis of predictive (prognostic) genetic information. Additionally, such legislation would stop both employers and insurers from requiring applicants to submit to genetic tests, maintain strict use and disclosure requirements of genetic test information, and impose penalties against employers and insurers who violate these provisions. Many states have enacted similar laws and some large employers have enacted their own policies to protect employees from discrimination. It is clear that all humans have genetic "flaws" and that our society is moving toward a more comfortable relationship with genetic information.

Heart structure in HCM

The normal heart (Figures 7 and 8)

First, it is helpful to be familiar with the structure and function of the normal heart in order to understand the abnormalities which occur in HCM. A normal heart has four heart chambers (left and right ventricles as the lower chambers; left and right atria as the upper chambers) and four valves (mitral and tricuspid; aortic and pulmonic). The walls of the heart are composed of muscle cells (myocytes), as well as collagen and small veins and arteries (called venules and arterioles, respectively). The left ventricular wall is normally about 3 times thicker than the right ventricle. The left

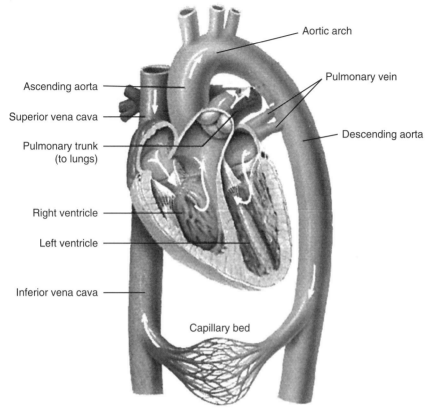

Aortic arch

Pulmonary vein

Ascending aorta

Superior vena cava

Descending aorta

Pulmonary trunk
(to lungs)

Right ventricle

Left ventricle

Inferior vena cava

Capillary bed

Figure 7 *Normal heart structure and blood flow.* It is helpful to be familiar with the structure and function of the normal heart in order to understand the abnormalities in HCM. This drawing shows a normal heart with heart chambers, valves, and the direction of blood flow. The walls of the heart are composed of specialized muscle known as the *myocardium*. The arrows show the direction of blood flow through the heart. The right atrium receives blood from the body, transfers it to the right ventricle which pumps it into the lungs to receive oxygen. This oxygenated blood returns to the heart from the lungs into the left atrium and is transferred to the left ventricle (through the mitral valve) which then pumps it into the systemic circulation.

ventricular wall is usually of similar thickness in all areas, and in normal adults measures 12 mm or less on the echocardiogram (in the relaxation phase – i.e., diastole).

The normal course of blood flow through the heart is shown in Figure 7. Every normal heartbeat results from an electrical signal which starts in the right atrium (sinoatrial node) and passes down through the conducting system of the heart and into the ventricles; the contraction of the heart follows the same sequence.

The heart in HCM (Figures 8–11)

In HCM, the left ventricular wall is abnormal by virtue of excessive thickening, while the cavity of the left ventricle is of normal or small size. HCM has often been referred to as an "enlarged heart," but is probably more accurately regarded as a "thickened" or "muscular" heart. The distribution of this muscle thickening (or hypertrophy) may take many forms

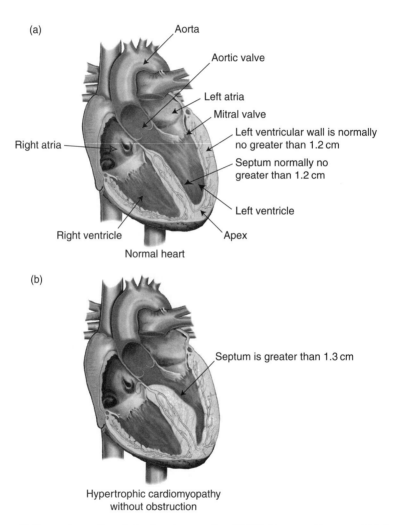

(a)

Aorta

Aortic valve

Left atria

Mitral valve

Left ventricular wall is normally no greater than 1.2 cm

Septum normally no greater than 1.2 cm

Right atria

Left ventricle

Right ventricle

Apex

Normal heart

(b)

Septum is greater than 1.3 cm

Hypertrophic cardiomyopathy without obstruction

Figure 8 *Comparison of heart structure in normal and HCM.* Compared to normal (a), the HCM heart (b) typically shows thickening of the ventricular septum which is greater than other parts of the left ventricular wall, whether or not obstruction is present.

(c)

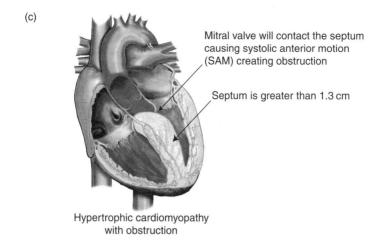

Mitral valve will contact the septum causing systolic anterior motion (SAM) creating obstruction

Septum is greater than 1.3 cm

Hypertrophic cardiomyopathy
with obstruction

Figure 8 (*continued*) However, the exact pattern of hypertrophy in HCM can be quite diverse and is not limited to that shown here. (c) The mechanism by which obstruction occurs when the mitral valve comes forward and contacts the septum (arrow) – that is, systolic anterior motion of the mitral valve (or SAM).

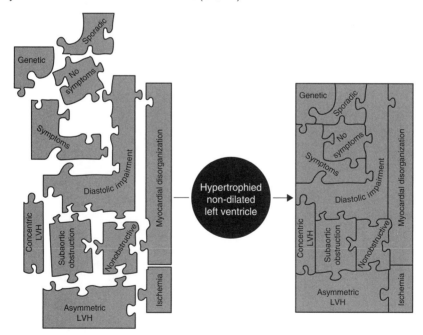

Figure 9 The clinical definition of HCM is based on the presence of left ventricular hypertrophy (LVH) without cavity enlargement … in a patient who does not have another cardiac (or systemic) disease that itself could potentially produce the degree of hypertrophy evident in that patient. This is the basic criterion for diagnosis that brings together the diverse jigsaw puzzle … that HCM often appears to be.

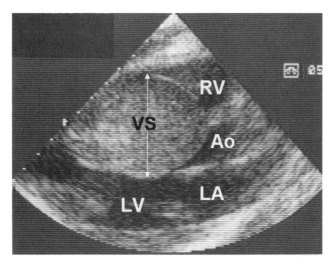

Figure 10 A stop-frame photograph from a two-dimensional echocardiogram of an HCM heart with extreme thickening of the left ventricular (LV) wall. Note that the ventricular septum (VS) measures 52 mm in thickness which is about 5 times normal. Ao: aorta; LA: left atrium; RV: right ventricle.

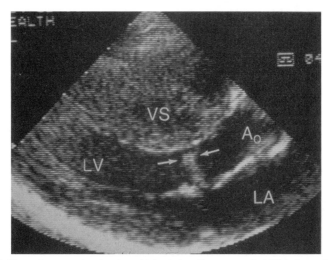

Figure 11 The unique mechanism by which obstruction occurs in HCM shown in a stop-frame echocardiogram. Note how a portion of the mitral valve comes forward to ultimately contact the thick ventricular septum (VS) (denoted by the arrows). Ao: aorta; LA: left atrium; LV: left ventricle cavity.

and differ greatly from patient to patient (even among related patients). The particular pattern, precise site, or degree of hypertrophy may vary considerably among patients, but can be of significance in selected individuals.

In addition, the absolute thickness of the wall may vary greatly among patients as well. HCM may reach thicknesses that far exceed that reported in any other cardiac disease – ranging up to 6 times normal. The upper limit of normal wall thickness is 10–12 mm and, remarkably, some patients may show thicknesses as much as 40–60 mm (Figure 10). Patients are often very focused on their exact "number" for wall thickness, but actually in most patients this precise value is of little significance. One exception would be those with an extremely thick wall of more than 30 or 35 mm for which increased risk for sudden death has been associated. On the other hand, many patients have only mildly increased thickness which may be confined to only a small portion of the left ventricular wall.

Usually, hypertrophy in HCM is described as **asymmetric** which means some parts of the wall are thicker than others (Figures 8 and 10). It is usually the ventricular septum which is thickest, and portions of the left ventricular free wall (i.e., not part of the septum) are usually thinner. The term "concentric" only means that all portions of the wall are the same thickness; this pattern of hypertrophy is uncommon in HCM, and present in only about 2% of patients.

HCM is a complex disease, and this point is underscored by the fact that a few adult individuals may harbor a gene defect for HCM but nevertheless have normal echocardiograms and electrocardiograms, and therefore would completely escape clinical recognition. Indeed, this is an example of *HCM without hypertrophy*, which can be diagnosed only with genetic testing. However, based on available information, there does not seem to be significant risk associated with this expression of HCM, although some of these individuals may "convert" to a more typical appearance of HCM in mid-life by developing a thick heart wall.

Other very different heart conditions may mimic HCM by virtue of showing a thickened heart, and the distinction may be difficult at times. These include diseases that infiltrate the heart (and other organs) like amyloidosis, which occurs almost exclusively in older patients, as well as other genetic conditions such as glycogen storage diseases, Noonan syndrome (in infants and young children) and Fabry's disease (in adults), and occasionally extreme examples of the benign "athlete's heart" … in which an increased thickness of the left ventricular wall is due solely to intense and chronic sports training.

Outflow obstruction

Muscle thickening involving the upper portion of ventricular septum is often associated with a unique motion pattern of the mitral valve (Figures 8c and 11). In such cases, during the ejection of the blood from the left ventricle (in systole) the mitral valve moves forward and contacts the septum (there should normally be a considerable gap between these two structures) and obstructs the outflow of blood from the left side of the heart into the aorta, thereby creating a *pressure gradient* between the aorta and left ventricle (Figures 8–11). Consequently, **left ventricular outflow obstruction** in HCM is actually caused by unique mitral valve motion and *not* due to the thickened septum, *per se*.

There is often considerable confusion among patients on this point … who may occasionally receive the mistaken impression that they have valve disease. The turbulent blood flow produced by obstruction creates a *murmur* – a sound that is audible with a stethoscope. Also, the abnormal mitral valve motion will cause blood to leak backward into the left atrium, called *mitral regurgitation*. Together, obstruction and mitral regurgitation cause the pressures within the chamber of the left ventricle to increase, which in turn adversely affects heart function.

Outflow obstruction, although present in the resting state (such as when you are having your echocardiogram performed) in about 25% of HCM patients, also commonly occurs with physical exertion and can account (with mitral regurgitation) for symptoms such as shortness of breath, fatigue, chest pain, and fainting which typically occur with activity. It was formerly believed that obstruction was relatively uncommon among HCM patients because only a minority has this finding under resting conditions. However, more recent data obtained by exercising patients on the treadmill show that a large number who have no obstruction at rest do in fact develop considerable gradients (i.e., obstruction) under normal physiologic exercise conditions. Therefore, it is now evident that fully 70% of all HCM patients have some obstruction either at rest … or with exercise.

The descriptive term – *obstruction* – often conveys a strong connotation to patients which may not always be entirely deserved. This word refers, of course, to only *partial* obstruction (or impedance) to the flow of blood from the left ventricle to aorta. Furthermore, the presence of obstruction is not always unfavorable to patients, and can be tolerated for many years with no or few symptoms. On the other hand, in some patients, severe limiting symptoms and disability can be attributed directly to the presence of obstruction (Figure 12).

Obstruction literally means the *difference* in pressure between the left ventricle and aorta measured in millimeters of mercury (i.e. mmHg). This

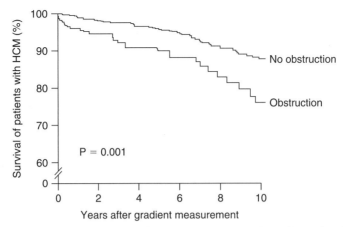

Figure 12 Comparison of survival of HCM patients with and without obstruction. Over long periods of time, obstruction conveys a significant risk (i.e., decrease in survival) due mostly to heart failure.

measurement is most commonly made non-invasively with routine Doppler echocardiography, or much less frequently with cardiac catheterization by determining pressure measurements directly with catheters introduced into the heart through arm vessels or through the groin. It is also important for patients to realize that obstruction in HCM may change spontaneously in degree – from day to day, hour to hour, with exercise or emotion, or even after a heavy meal or consumption of a small amount of alcohol. Therefore, patients should consider the actual numerical value for the gradient obtained at any given time in light of this dynamic nature and potential change, and not necessarily as a fixed number. Patients often become overly concerned about their "gradient-number" (particularly if it is perceived as large or increasing), but are advised to keep these points in mind and to discuss the true significance of their gradient in their specific case with their cardiologist.

Heart function in HCM

The thickened muscle of the left ventricle in HCM usually contracts well in the presence of small- or normal-sized heart chambers – sometimes even better than normal – and rapidly ejects most of the blood from the heart (i.e., in systole). There are no particular adverse or beneficial implications to having a ventricle that contracts in this way. Only a very few HCM patients develop depressed contraction associated with severe heart failure (as will be discussed later). However, the heart muscle in HCM is often stiff and relaxes poorly when blood enters the ventricles passively during diastole (i.e., relaxation). It is believed that symptoms in HCM (such as shortness of breath with exercise) can be related, at least in part, to this impaired filling of the ventricles or obstruction. Therefore, the type of "heart failure" characteristic of HCM in which the heart actually contracts normally is very different from the much more common situation (due to coronary heart disease and heart attacks, or long-standing high blood pressure), in which there is usually abnormal enlargement of the ventricles and impaired contraction.

Ischemia – impaired blood flow to the heart muscle – may also be responsible for symptoms (including chest pain) in HCM, and may have unfavorable consequences because it can cause heart cells to die and be replaced by scars. In this regard, ischemia in HCM is similar to that experienced by patients with coronary artery disease due to atherosclerosis (with plaques in the large coronary arteries). HCM patients with ischemia may have either true angina pectoris (relatively short-lasting pain or pressure in the center of the chest associated with exertion or occurring after meals) or "atypical" pain patterns that differ from classic angina in a variety of ways.

However, in HCM, ischemia occurs by a different mechanism than in coronary heart disease, and probably results from abnormal function of small arteries *within* the heart muscle which have thickened walls and narrowed openings. It is also possible that this ischemia results in part because the heart muscle is too thick for the available blood supply. Unfortunately, identifying ischemia in HCM with routinely available tests is difficult and often unreliable; positron emission tomography (PET) can be useful in this regard – but is generally not available for routine testing. Therefore, it has been challenging to assess this particular problem with precision in HCM patients.

When does HCM develop?: HCM in infants and children

Since HCM is a genetic disease, the mutant gene is (of course) present from conception and all affected family members carry exactly the same mutation. While hypertrophy, as visualized with the echocardiogram, may occasionally be present at birth or in very young children, it is actually much more common for the heart to appear normal until about age 12 years in genetically affected family members. Usually hypertrophy then develops in association with accelerated growth and is apparent on the echocardiogram in the teenage years by about age 13–14 years. Although the vast majority of patients do not show significant change in muscle thickness after age 18 years, we now know that it is also possible for the heart to thicken at virtually any age. This phenomenon of "late-onset" hypertrophy has been observed in mid-life and even beyond, but its frequency is unknown (and will be discussed later).

HCM is identified uncommonly in children and therefore is regarded as a rare disease by pediatric cardiologists. Most children diagnosed with HCM are initially suspected by either a heart murmur, transient symptoms, abnormal ECG, or family history of HCM. On occasion, this suspicion may arise during preparticipation screening for competitive athletics – and is confirmed later by echocardiography.

The proportion of HCM children with important and limiting symptoms is small, and the occurrence of sudden unexpected death before age 10 years appears to be exceedingly uncommon. Nevertheless, occasionally HCM may be detected in young children. Most often this occurs fortuitously (by a chance occurrence) when a murmur is heard – in a healthy-appearing child, or during routine family screening. There are probably no particular long-term consequences attached to HCM should it be discovered at a young age in this way. However, when symptoms of heart failure have a very early onset in life, and/or hypertrophy is substantial, these findings may well connote a more severe form of the disease. At present, specific data on this point are sparse.

Indeed, the diagnosis of HCM in children and adolescents often represents a major dilemma for pediatric cardiologists since the patients are young and predictions regarding future prognosis are therefore much more difficult. It is possible for such circumstances to lead to over-reaction and there is occasionally a tendency to pursue major interventions … perhaps prematurely. On the other hand, there may also be some reticence to initiate chronic device therapy (e.g., implantable defibrillators or pacemakers) because of the youthful age and healthy appearance, lack of symptoms, and active lifestyle.

Very rarely, HCM presents during infancy with heart failure; this appears to be a particularly unfavorable development and many of these children die early in life despite aggressive drug therapy. However, of note, most infants or young children (<4 years) with thick hearts may not have traditional HCM. Often a number of other diverse conditions occur in which the heart manifestations can mimic HCM (most commonly Noonan syndrome and glycogen storage diseases), or when diabetes is present in the mother during pregnancy – a situation in which the hypertrophy in the newborn may quickly disappear spontaneously within a few weeks.

Gender and race

In published clinical papers HCM is always reported to be more common in men than in women (usually about 60:40 or 65:35). However, in reality, because HCM is a genetic disease transmitted as an autosomal dominant trait, it will occur equally in men and women. This means that HCM is *diagnosed* less frequently in women than men. The reason for this circumstance is uncertain. However, there is now evidence that women with HCM (compared to men) develop symptoms later in life, are diagnosed at more advanced ages, and in fact experience more severe heart failure.

HCM has always been uncommonly diagnosed in African-Americans in clinical settings. Paradoxically, previously unsuspected HCM has proved to be a common cause of sudden death in young black male athletes on the athletic field. This suggests that the rarity of an HCM diagnosis in young African-Americans is probably due largely to socioeconomic factors which create more limited access to the subspecialty medical establishment (which is a prerequisite for obtaining an echocardiogram and thereby an HCM diagnosis).

What are the symptoms of HCM?

It is important to realize that HCM is an unusual disease by virtue of affecting people at virtually any age. Patients from infancy (as young as the first day of life) to the elderly (as old as >90 years of age) may develop HCM-related symptoms. HCM symptoms are generally similar to that of other forms of heart disease and there is no particular complaint which is unique to this disease. Not uncommonly, patients may relate symptoms of shortness of breath or chest pain. Patients often relate "good and bad days" during which such symptoms may be perceived as quite different in degree. The precise basis for this variability is uncertain. However, when relating symptoms to your cardiologist it is important not to limit your history to either extreme (i.e., the best or worst), but rather provide the complete spectrum of complaints which you experience on a daily basis. It is particularly important to advise your cardiologist of any new or consistently increased symptoms.

Shortness of breath. Exercise capacity may be limited by shortness of breath and fatigue (also called exertional **dyspnea**). Most HCM patients experience only mild exercise limitation, but occasionally this becomes severe and patients are unable to walk even one city block at a reasonable pace, or a flight of stairs, without stopping due to shortness of breath; a minority may have shortness of breath at rest.

Chest pain. Chest pain or pressure (sometimes called *angina*) is a common symptom. It is usually brought on by exertion and relieved by rest, but may also occur at rest. In HCM, chest discomfort may also take different forms – sharp or dull, in the center of the chest or elsewhere, or prolonged and unrelated to exertion. The cause of the pain is thought to be insufficient oxygen supply to the heart muscle (**ischemia**). In HCM, the main coronary arteries are usually free of significant plaque or narrowing from atherosclerosis. However, in contrast, the smaller arteries well within the heart muscle are often narrowed; the greatly thickened left well ventricular muscle demands an increased oxygen supply which often cannot be served by the abnormal small arteries.

Fatigue. A complaint distinctive from shortness of breath with exertion; many patients complain of excessive tiredness, either related or unrelated to exertion, and the necessity to nap frequently.

Palpitations. Patients may occasionally feel an extra or skipped beat, and this may be normal and unrelated to HCM. Sometimes, however, such an awareness of the beating heart may be prolonged and indicative of an irregular heart rhythm. This symptom, **palpitations**, may also occur commonly in other forms of heart disease, and even frequently in people without any form of heart disease. Palpitations begin suddenly, and may be associated with symptoms such as sweating or lightheadedness. Such episodes should be reported to your cardiologist and investigated.

Lightheadedness, near-fainting, and fainting. Patients with HCM may experience impairment or loss of consciousness (i.e., lightheadedness or dizziness) and, more seriously, fainting (known as **syncope**) … or the perception that a loss of consciousness is imminent, but then does not in fact occur (**near-syncope**). Such episodes may occur in association with exercise, or without apparent provocation, and the reason for these events is not always clear, even after testing. Impaired consciousness may be due to an irregularity of the heartbeat, a fall in blood pressure, or very commonly unrelated to HCM and heart disease – "simple faint" or vasovagal syncope – in which the vagal nerve is excessively active. Fainting (or near-fainting) should be reported immediately to your cardiologist and investigated. Unfortunately, such episodes represent the most difficult HCM symptom to evaluate – simply because the events occur without warning and are over long before your physician can order tests to investigate their origin.

Mis-diagnosis

The HCMA has collected specific, clinical information from nearly 3,000 families living with HCM. It has become clear that there are patterns of mis-diagnosis with ties to age, gender, and geography. Forty percent of HCM patients had been initially diagnosed with a condition other than HCM, waiting as long as 35 years to obtain an accurate diagnosis. Children and adolescents may be incorrectly diagnosed with asthma … and frequently "exercise-induced asthma", particularly in athletes. This can be a troubling situation as some asthma medications (mainly albuterol containing inhalers) contain properties that may promote arrhythmias.

Men with HCM may be told they have depression, panic disorder, or "athlete's heart" when in fact their symptoms are directly linked to HCM. While depression and panic disorders are important diagnoses, it is possible to have these conditions as well as HCM. Women with HCM are often initially diagnosed with mitral valve prolapse, panic disorders, or an innocent murmur. Patients with HCM living in rural areas are diagnosed later, and face much longer periods of ambiguity, than those living in urban areas.

How is HCM diagnosed and what tests are used?

Physical examination. In many patients with HCM, the physical examination is unremarkable and either only a soft heart murmur or no murmur at all is heard. This fact is surprising to many people, but only reflects the fact that under resting conditions most HCM patients do not have obstruction to the flow of blood from the left ventricle (as discussed previously). This infrequency with which a loud heart murmur occurs accounts, in part, for the difficulty in identifying HCM during the routine preparticipation screening of competitive athletes.

Most HCM patients (particularly young people) have a prominant heart impulse that can be felt or even seen on the left side of the chest, and which reflects the thickened and forcibly contracting heart. This observation may trigger recognition of HCM in some instances, even in the absence of a loud heart murmur.

Indeed, when present, the most obvious finding on physical examination is a systolic heart murmur. Such murmurs usually indicate partial obstruction to blood flow out of the left side of the heart, and may change spontaneously throughout the day and with activity. Your cardiologist may also be able to provoke a heart murmur by asking you to change body position (i.e., stand) or undergo maneuvers such as holding your breath and straining (Valsalva), inhaling amyl nitrite, or exercising on a treadmill. However, in general, the presence of a heart murmur is not necessarily an unfavorable sign – it simply indicates the presence of obstruction and/or an insufficient mitral valve. While HCM may be suspected by findings on physical examination, this is not usually the way diagnosis is made.

Echocardiogram. The primary test for the clinical diagnosis of HCM is an ultrasound scan of the heart called an **echocardiogram**. This is an entirely safe non-invasive test which produces two-dimensional images of the heart which are viewed in real-time, and recorded along with single-dimensional views (called the derived M-mode echocardiogram). The echocardiogram is performed by a specially trained technologist (the cardiologist may or may not be present during the test) who places a transducer and a small amount of transmitting gel on the chest to generate images of the heart in several cross-sectional views (Figure 13a). The excessive thickness of the left ventricular wall in HCM is easily (and traditionally) measured from the echocardiographic images. An additional ultrasound mode called *Doppler* is very useful with regard to heart function and includes a color-coded image of blood flow within the heart. Turbulent flow and the degree of obstruction (if present), as well as valve leakage (mitral regurgitation), can be detected and measured with precision. Therefore, the echocardiogram can provide a thorough structural and functional assessment of HCM, largely avoiding invasive procedures such as cardiac catheterization. However is some rare case in specialized HCM centers catheterization may be used to access the level of obstruction if such measurements remain unclear based on non-invasive testing.

Electrocardiogram (ECG). The standard electrocardiogram (also known as the 12-lead ECG) is performed by placing electrodes on the chest, wrists, and ankles and recording the electrical signals from the heart. In HCM, the ECG usually shows a wide variety of abnormal electrical signals usually due to the muscle thickening. Alternatively, in a small minority of patients the ECG may be normal or show particularly minor alterations. The ECG abnormalities are not specific to HCM and may also

(a)

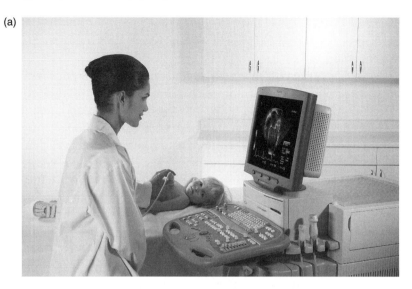

(b)

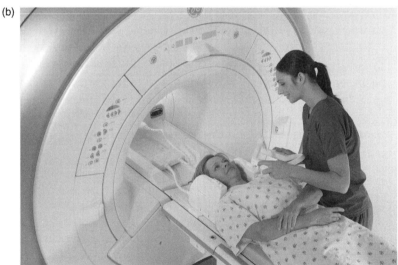

Figure 13 (a) The clinical diagnosis of HCM is generally made with imaging tests, most commonly with an ultrasound scan of the heart called an echocardiogram (or echo, for short) or alternatively with increasing frequency with cardiac magnetic resonance (MRI) (b). Both techniques are entirely safe and pain-free, and produce a number of images of the heart, so that excessive thickness of the heart muscle wall, characteristic of HCM, can be easily measured. MRI has the additional capacity to visualize areas of scarring within the wall and can more reliably identify hypertrophy in certain regions of the heart. At present, echocardiography is the primary diagnostic test, with MRI used selectively as a supplement. Photographs courtesy of GE Healthcare.

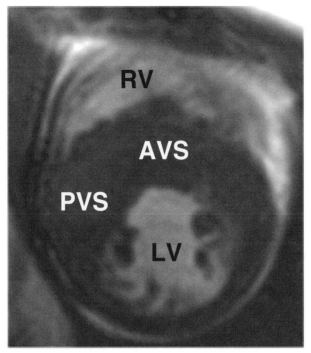

Figure 14 An MRI image of the heart in HCM. The left ventricle (LV) is visualized in cross-section and appears as a "donut". Note that the ventricular septum (designated AVS for anterior portion of ventricular septum and PVS for posterior ventricular septum) is much thicker than other parts of the wall. RV: right ventricle.

be found in many other heart conditions. In fact, the abnormal ECG in HCM can frequently mimic that of a previous, healed, myocardial infarction ("heart attack"). Indeed, some HCM patients have been advised erroneously that they have previously experienced a "heart attack." However, keep in mind that "heart attack" is a non-medical term which literally refers to sudden occurrences of heart damage due solely to the consequence of coronary artery disease with atherosclerosis.

Cardiac magnetic resonance (MRI) (Figure 13b). While two-dimensional echocardiography is the primary clinical test to diagnose HCM, MRI based on magnet technology, may provide extremely high-quality images of the heart which are often superior to echocardiography. MRI may provide diagnostic images of the heart and more precise measurement of wall thickness when the echocardiogram is ambiguous or not of sufficient technical quality (Figure 14). Furthermore, of note, in selected patients MRI may in fact image thick areas of the left ventricular wall which are not accessible to conventional echocardiography. Therefore, MRI may be the only imaging test capable of making the diagnosis of HCM in a few patients. In addition, MRI provides the opportunity to visualize scar formation (i.e., fibrosis) within the wall of the left ventricle by virtue of the injection of a compound called gadolinium during the study (Figure 13b). However, particularly obese patients and those with claustrophobia may not be suitable candidates for MRI. Your cardiologist may elect to perform an MRI in addition to the echocardiogram for any of the aforementioned reasons.

Genetic testing. Laboratory DNA analysis (of blood or other tissue) is, of course, the most definitive method for making the diagnosis of HCM. Previously, most successful genotyping had been achieved through selected participation in a research project. However, a genetic test for HCM diagnosis (requiring 7 ml of blood) is now available commercially (see Appendix). This procedure tests the 10 most common genes causing the disease and provides results in about 4–6 weeks. The test is expensive ($5,650 for 10 genes) and at this time must be negotiated on a case-by-case basis with insurance companies and also harbors a significant likelihood of "false-negative" test results (in which the test cannot detect a mutant gene for HCM because that gene is one of the many which have not yet been identified). However, if the family mutation is known, other relatives can be tested definitively for $250 each.

Other investigations that may be useful

Additional investigations may be required in selected patients to assess HCM.

Cardiac catheterization. Due to the widespread use of non-invasive imaging with echocardiography, Doppler, and MRI, there is no longer a compelling reason to perform cardiac catheterization procedures to evaluate HCM. However, because it is possible for HCM patients over age 40 years (with or without a history of chest pain) to also have coronary artery disease, it may be necessary in some circumstances to perform a cardiac catheterization with angiography to define the anatomy of the coronary arteries. Most recently, computed tomography angiograms have become available, which can non-invasively screen the coronary arteries for narrowings.

With *cardiac catheterization*, a fine tube is passed through a vein (usually in the groin) to the heart using X-ray guidance. Pressures within the heart chambers are then measured, and an *angiogram* (X-ray) of the heart can be obtained by the injection of contrast dye to assess an incompetent mitral valve (mitral regurgitation), contraction of the left ventricle, or narrowing of the coronary arteries by arterosclerotic plaque.

Electrophysiological studies. This is a specialized form of cardiac catheterization which has been performed selectively to define the risk of electrical instability which may predispose to sudden death. *Electrophysiological studies* involve the passage of fine wires from the veins in the groin, arm, or shoulder into the heart under X-ray guidance. These wires are then used to make measurements or apply stimuli to record the response of the electrical system of the heart. Sometimes irregularities of the heartbeat (otherwise known as **arrhythmia**) are intentionally provoked in the laboratory (and immediately terminated) to estimate a patient's predisposition to develop such rhythms naturally. At present, most investigators believe that electrophysiologic testing is not particularly informative for assessing risk for sudden death in HCM patients.

Exercise testing. The severity of exercise limitation and the effect of treatment can be assessed with bicycle or treadmill *exercise testing*. Exercise testing can also provide an objective measurement of improvement, stability, or deterioration over time. Of note, the exercise test is often combined with an echocardiogram (stress echocardiogram) to determine whether outflow obstruction occurs physiologically with exertion. This particular test is used with increasing frequency on a routine basis since knowledge of such provoked obstruction may have clinical relevance … that is, replicate the circumstances under which patients experience exertion-related symptoms. If you have limiting shortness of breath, but no obstruction at rest, your cardiologist may want to perform a stress echocardiogram to determine whether you develop obstruction while engaged in physical activity which produces symptoms. This may allow you to become a candidate for a potentially beneficial treatment intervention, such as myectomy surgery, or alcohol septal ablation (in very selected patients). Also, blood pressure drop or its failure to increase appropriately during exercise in some patients may indicate an important instability and are currently identified as a potential risk factor.

Ambulatory Holter monitoring. This test is a non-invasive and continuous recording of the heartbeat over 24 or 48 hours during normal activities. A Holter monitor is a simple test that will detect potentially important irregularities of the heartbeat of which the patient is usually unaware.

Radionuclide studies. In these tests, substances producing very tiny (safe) amounts of radioactivity are injected into the bloodstream to create a heart scan. These tests are occasionally performed in HCM patients to assess the contraction and filling of the ventricles, at rest and with exercise.

General outlook for patients with HCM

The severity of symptoms and risk of complications vary greatly between HCM patients, and it should be emphasized that many individuals never experience serious problems related to their disease. Indeed, HCM may not reduce life expectancy and is compatible with normal longevity. It is not unusual for patients to be in their 70s and 80s, including even some patients who have survived into their 90s … and without significant disability, limitation in quality of life, or the need to undergo major treatment interventions to achieve these goals. When considering the *overall* adult population with HCM, this disease may not add significantly to individual risk – over the known risks of living, such as those related to cancer, diabetes, coronary heart disease, or accidents, etc. (Figures 15 and 16). The most accurate mortality rate characterizing the overall disease is about 1% per year, which means that each year no more than 1 of 100 patients may die for any reason.

On the other hand, many patients experience significant symptoms, disability, or may be at risk for premature death. There are three circumstances in which patients with HCM die prematurely: (1) suddenly and unexpectedly, most commonly in younger patients; (2) related to severe progressive heart failure, usually in mid-life; and (3) due to stroke, generally in older patients with atrial fibrillation. Limiting symptoms (i.e., shortness of breath and/or chest pain with exertion) may remain stable and controlled for many years, or deteriorate and require a major intervention. However, each patient with HCM must be assessed individually to determine which subgroup of patients they most likely belong – for example, high or low risk for sudden death … and with or without predisposition to progressive symptoms or atrial fibrillation.

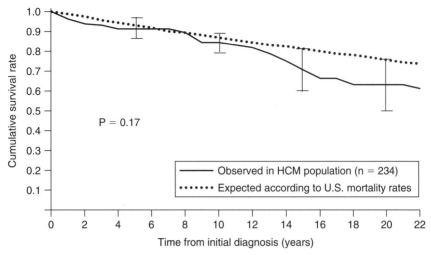

Figure 15 Survival in a regional HCM population from the upper Mid-West compared to that in the general U.S. population (mortality due to all causes; e.g., cancer, homicide, coronary heart disease, etc.). The two populations are not different in terms of survival. *Therefore, HCM itself does not add to the overall risk of living.*

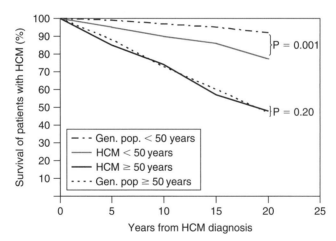

Figure 16 Survival curves of HCM patients compared to that of the general population (gen. pop.) including all the risks of living. For HCM patients diagnosed at age 50 years or older, the life expectancy is the same as for the general population.

Therefore, it is an important general principle regarding HCM ... that all patients are *not* the same in terms of prognosis, clinical presentation, nor potential treatment options (Figure 17). Since there are several different clinical profiles that patients may adopt, it is important not to "lump" all

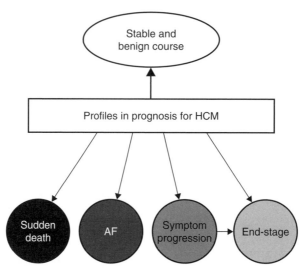

Figure 17 *Profiles in prognosis*. Most patients with HCM can be placed in one of these categories for the purposes of judging prognosis, as well as eventually formulating treatment strategies. This diagram emphasizes the necessity of viewing HCM in terms of such subgroups so that treatment can be tailored to a particular clinical profile. However, not all patients have these complications, as many experience a benign and stable course. AF: atrial fibrillation.

patients together under the homogeneous label of HCM. Indeed, while some patients have little or no risk associated with their disease, others deserve high-risk status. *However, the overall disease is not*, per se, *high risk, and HCM should not be regarded as a uniformly unfavorable condition.* Obviously, this book provides only a broad overview of prognosis for HCM patients and cannot substitute for the careful evaluation of an individual patient by a cardiologist knowledgeable about this disease.

Complications of HCM

Arrhythmias

A variety of arrhythmias (irregularities of the heartbeat) are exceedingly common in patients with HCM and can be detected by Holter monitoring, exercise testing, or ECG. Prolonged arrhythmias known as *ventricular tachycardia* or *atrial fibrillation* are particularly important and require treatment in the vast majority of cases. Transient arrhythmias with premature beats originating from the atria and ventricles occur much more commonly, but usually do not have particular clinical importance to patients, even when present in large numbers.

Ventricular tachycardia/ventricular fibrillation. Ventricular tachycardia is an incessant and repetitive occurrence of abnormal beats arising from the ventricles. This is a potentially serious arrhythmia in HCM since it may lead to ventricular fibrillation and sudden death. Patients prone to these arrhythmias may be treated with an implantable cardioverter-defibrillator, designed to sense and automatically terminate these arrhythmias (as will be discussed later).

Atrial fibrillation and stroke. With atrial fibrillation, the normal regular heart rhythm is altered due to loss of the contraction of the atria (the two upper chambers), causing the ventricles to beat in an irregular rhythm. Atrial fibrillation may be episodic (i.e., paroxysmal) or persistent (i.e., chronic), occurs in as much as 20–25% of HCM patients, is often responsible for important symptoms of heart failure, but does not appear to be specifically associated with an increased risk for sudden cardiac death. While some patients are unaware of their atrial fibrillation, most rapidly develop symptoms such as shortness of breath, dizziness, and fainting. Atrial fibrillation increases in frequency with age, but may occur at any time in adulthood (usually after about age 30–35 years). It is much less common for atrial fibrillation to occur in younger patients.

Because the atria "fibrillate" there is risk for clot formation due to stagnant blood flow. This can result in a stroke if the blood clot travels to the brain. The risk of such an event is about 1% per year in HCM patients with atrial fibrillation. Anticoagulation, to protect against stroke, is an important consideration, and the pros and cons of this treatment should be discussed in detail with your cardiologist.

Sometimes atrial fibrillation will revert to normal rhythm spontaneously, but patients often require drug treatment to abolish the abnormal rhythm or control and reduce the rapid ventricular rate (if the patient must remain in atrial fibrillation). However, *electrical cardioversion* may be used to convert the heart back into its normal rhythm. This treatment requires admission to the hospital and consists of applying an electrical shock to the chest, often following a course of anticoagulant medication. Atrial fibrillation also occurs in forms of heart disease other than HCM (and also in patients without heart disease, i.e. "lone atrial fibrillation"). Other emerging treatments for atrial fibrillation in HCM and other diseases include The MAZE procedure, in which the electrical connection in the left atria is interrupted at surgery (often performed at the time of myectomy in HCM). Also, radio frequency ablation is a non-surgical procedure performed via a catheter, in which the abnormal electrical pathway is interrupted to terminate the conduction of extra impulses which create rapid heartbeats and atrial fibrillation. The overall effectiveness of either strategy, in HCM, is currently unresolved, and at an early stage of development.

Heart failure

Any HCM patient with significant shortness of breath during physical exertion is, strictly speaking, experiencing a degree of heart failure. However, this is a different form of heart failure than occurs in patients with coronary artery disease, or many other cardiac conditions. In HCM, heart failure is paradoxically present in a heart which is not dilated and actually shows normal contraction of the ventricles. In other more common diseases, congestive heart failure is usually a profound condition, generally occurring after a myocardial infarction ("heart attack"), and producing dilated ventricles that contract poorly. Occasionally, heart failure in HCM may become intractable and fail to respond to drugs, requiring major intervention and treatment, such as with surgical myectomy (alcohol septal ablation is a selective alternative), or very occasionally heart transplant.

The problem of sudden death

Since the first description of HCM almost 50 years ago, the issue of risk for sudden and unexpected death has been a highly visible issue. However, it should be emphasized that in reality only a small proportion of patients with HCM are at increased risk for sudden premature death due to arrhythmias (Figure 18). Also, the magnitude of this problem of sudden death has probably been exaggerated over the years due to the disproportionate number of reports from institutions in which there was the preferential referral of high-risk patients (i.e., the so-called tertiary centers).

Nevertheless, sudden unexpected collapse remains a devastating consideration for many patients living with this disease. There are no reliable clinical warning signs and therefore the assignment of high-risk status is not dependent on, for example, the prior occurrences of fainting or other symptoms. We know that sudden death occurs most commonly in young

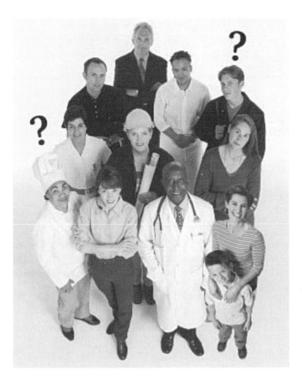

Figure 18 While the risk for sudden death in young people has been a highly visible feature of HCM, in reality it is an uncommon occurrence and only a minority of patients are truly at risk. Therefore, an important aspiration of the HCM evaluation is to identify which specific patients, among all those with this condition, are at high risk.

people (under 30–35 years old), but on the other hand there is no particular age which is completely immune, and sudden deaths due to HCM have been reported in mid-life and beyond. The first 10–12 years of life are generally, but not invariably, free of adverse events (at a time when it is also uncommon for hypertrophy to have appeared). Only a few early onset cases of young children with substantial hypertrophy or sudden death have been reported.

Sudden death may occur in some susceptible patients with HCM because the abnormal heart muscle can sometimes interfere with normal electrical activity (i.e., cause electrical instability). For example, in those portions of the left ventricular wall with abnormal architecture and cell disarray, the electrical signal may become unstable as it crosses areas of scarring and disorganized cells (Figures 1 and 19). This can, in turn, lead

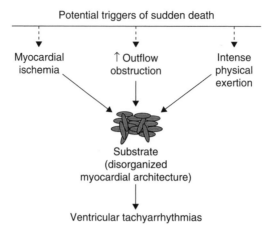

Potential triggers of sudden death

Myocardial ischemia ↑ Outflow obstruction Intense physical exertion

Substrate (disorganized myocardial architecture)

Ventricular tachyarrhythmias

Figure 19 Proposed mechanism by which myocardial disarray (as the electrically unstable "substrate") may promote serious ventricular arrhythmias ... when activated by a variety of (largely undefined) "triggers" that may either be part of the HCM disease process or environmental factors such as intense physical exertion.

to distorted electrical impulses that generate fast or erratic heart rhythms, some of which can result in adverse clinical events.

A patient's risk for sudden death is judged by the presence or absence of certain disease features (i.e., "risk factors"). At present, the highest risk for sudden death appears to be associated with one or more of the following six risk factors (Figure 20): (1) prior cardiac arrest (complete heart stoppage); (2) fainting, particularly when repetitive or associated with exertion, or when occurring in young people; (3) serious arrhythmias (such as ventricular tachycardia) repeatedly detected by ambulatory Holter ECG monitoring; (4) a drop, or failure to rise, in blood pressure during exercise; (5) family history of HCM-related premature sudden death in one or more close relatives; or (6) extreme increase in the thickness of the left ventricular wall, particularly in young patients. The latter disease feature applies to about 10% of all HCM patients in whom the maximum thickness of the left ventricular wall is 3.0 cm (30 mm) or more and who may be at increased risk based solely on their particular heart structure (Figures 10 and 21).

In this regard, the term "risk stratification" is used to describe those tests, symptoms, and disease characteristics which are conventionally used to determine if a given patient should be regarded as at "high risk" for sudden cardiac arrest. Patients with one or more risk factors are encouraged to discuss ICD therapy with their cardiologist. Unfortunately, we know that

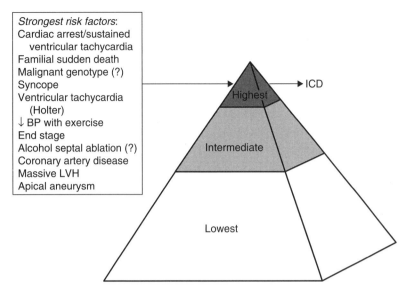

Strongest risk factors:
Cardiac arrest/sustained
    ventricular tachycardia
Familial sudden death
Malignant genotype (?)
Syncope
Ventricular tachycardia
    (Holter)
↓ BP with exercise
End stage
Alcohol septal ablation (?)
Coronary artery disease
Massive LVH
Apical aneurysm

ICD

Highest

Intermediate

Lowest

Figure 20 *The HCM disease features which give a patient high-risk status.* The presence of one or more of these clinical risk factors is sufficient to assign high-risk status and justify consideration for treatment to prevent sudden death, with an implantable cardioverter-defibrillator (ICD). ↓ BP = decreased blood pressure; LVH = left ventricular hypertrophy.

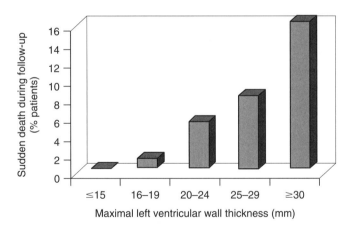

Figure 21 *Relation between the degree to which the left ventricular wall is thickened and the likelihood of sudden death.* This analysis shows that little risk is associated with mild degrees of thickening, while extreme increase in wall thickness (≥30 mm) conveys much greater risk. Therefore, the presence of extreme hypertrophy is risk factor for sudden death in HCM.

occasionally patients with none of the known risk factors may also suffer cardiac arrest.

On the other hand, and deserving of equal emphasis, most patients with HCM are without risk factors for sudden death, are at low risk for premature death, and therefore are deserving of a large measure of reassurance in this regard. Indeed, patients identified in adulthood have the same subsequent life expectancy as the general U.S. population.

Endocarditis

Endocarditis is an infection of the heart which occurs very uncommonly in HCM. Nevertheless, it is important to be protected from the unlikely disease complication since severe tissue damage of the heart valve can result, sometimes necessitating surgical replacement. Bacteria which gain access to the bloodstream can stick to the inside of the heart (specifically, on the mitral valve) after it has been roughened by turbulent blood flow. The risk of bacterial endocarditis in HCM seems to be largely limited to those patients with the obstructive form.

Aneurysms in HCM

An extraordinarily small proportion of HCM patients (about 1%) may develop a relatively small area of the left ventricle at its tip in which the wall bulges outward due to thinning with scarring. These aneurysms are important because they can be the source of serious arrhythmias, and may justify placement of an implantable defibrillator to prevent sudden death. However, there is no evidence at present that these aneurysms can rupture, and there is also little information available regarding whether they enlarge, or if so, at what rate. The aneurysm is identified best with MRI, but if large it can also be easily imaged with echocardiography. The mechanism by which this particular abnormality forms is completely unknown.

End-stage phase

This part of the HCM disease spectrum is also discussed later in more detail within the section on heart transplantation … to which it is linked clinically. The end stage is characterized by a change in the structure and function of the left ventricle due to gradual scarring which ultimately results in poor contractility and enlargement of the cavity and progressive heart failure.

Special considerations: Athletes and sports activities

While sudden death is very uncommon among all HCM patients ... HCM is, on the other hand, the most frequent cause of sudden cardiac death in young people (Figures 22 and 23), including participants in high school and

(a)

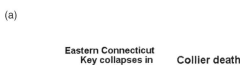

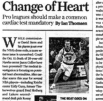

(b) "The time you won your town the race
We chaired you through the market-place;
Man and boy stood cheering by,
And home we brought you shoulder high.

To-day, the road all runners come,
Shoulder-high we bring you home,
And set you at your threshold down,
Townsman of a stiller town."

To An Athlete Dying Young
Alfred Edward Housmann, 1859

Figure 22 (a) Athletic field deaths in young sports participants have achieved a high level of public visibility in the news media. HCM is the single most common cause of these deaths. (b) A 110-year old poem which reflects a public perception of athlete sudden deaths ... true even to this day.

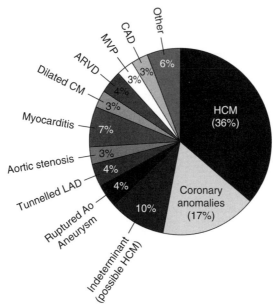

Figure 23 *Sudden death in young trained athletes.* HCM accounts for about one-third of these tragic events. Several other (mostly congenital) forms of heart disease shown are less commonly responsible for deaths in young athletes. Ao: aorta; ARVD: arrhythmogenic right ventricular dysplasia; AS: aortic stenosis; CAD: coronary artery disease (due to atherosclerosis); CM: cardiomyopathy; LAD: left anterior descending coronary artery; MVP: mitral valve prolapse.

college competitive sports. While HCM is responsible for one-third of such deaths, several other congenital disorders also result in such catastrophes. Based on these observations, it seems most prudent to withdraw young people from intense competitive sports when the diagnosis of HCM is made in order to lower risk. This applies to most organized athletic activities, particularly those involving exertion for which heart rate increases abruptly. Alternatively, participation in a few low-intensity competitive sports, such as golf and bowling are more acceptable. It is largely accepted that competitive athletics, or any lifestyle consistently involving intense physical exertion, adds to the risk of serious consequences from HCM – and removal from such activities will restore that individual to a more acceptable risk level. Indeed, removal of athletes with HCM from organized competitive sports can itself be regarded as a potentially beneficial treatment strategy.

National recommendations concerning criteria for sports eligibility and disqualification with cardiovascular disease have been formalized in a document known as *Bethesda Conference #36*, sponsored by the American College of Cardiology and published in the *Journal of the American College of*

Table 1 Recommendations regarding physical activity and recreational (non-competitive) sports participation for young patients with HCM*. Reproduced with permission from the American Heart Association.

Intensity level	HCM†	Intensity level	HCM†
High		*Moderate (cont.)*	
Basketball		Motorcycling§	3
Full court	0	Jogging	3
Half court	0	Sailingα	3
Body building§	1	Surfingα	2
Ice hockey§	0	Swimming (lap)α	5
Gymnastics	2	Tennis (doubles)	4
Racquetball/squash	0	Treadmill/stationary bicycle	5
Rock climbing§	1	Weightlifting (free weights)§¶	1
Running (sprinting)	0	Hiking	3
Skiing (downhill)§	2		
Skiing (cross-country)	2	*Low*	
Soccer	0	Bowling	5
Tennis (singles)	0	Golf	5
Touch (flag) football	1	Horseback riding§	3
Windsurfingα	1	Scuba divingα	0
		Skating (non-hockey)	5
Moderate		Snorkelingα	5
Baseball/softball	2	Weights (non-free weights)	4
Biking	4	Brisk walking	5
Modest hiking	4		

* Recreational sports are categorized with regard to high, moderate, and low levels of exercise and graded on a relative scale (from 0 to 5) for eligibility with 0 to 1 indicating *generally not advised or strongly discouraged*; 4 to 5 indicating *probably permitted*; and 2 to 3 indicating intermediate (and to be assessed clinically on an individual basis).

† Assumes absence of laboratory DNA genotyping and, therefore, limited to a clinical diagnosis.

§ These sports involve the potential for traumatic injury, which should be taken into consideration for individuals with a risk for impaired consciousness.

α The possibility of syncope occurring during water-related activities should be taken into account with respect to the clinical profile of the individual patient.

¶ Recommendations are generally more flexible for the use of weight-training machines (i.e., for non-free weights).

Cardiology in 2005. Young patients with HCM often wish to exercise and participate in recreational physical activities, whether or not they have personally been active in competitive sports. Such recommendations to patients are often complex. However, a recent American Heart Association document is available, offering specific recommendations for a variety of activities in genetic heart diseases such as HCM. A portion of this document is reproduced in Table 1. The guidelines recommend avoiding recreational sports that involve:

1 "Burst" (sprinting) exertion with rapid acceleration and deceleration (and abrupt change in heart rate) over short distances.

2 Adverse environmental conditions including particularly cold or hot (and humid) temperatures.

3 Systematic and progressive levels of exertion and training focused on achieving higher levels of conditioning and excellence.

4 Excessive or prolonged participation in sports otherwise intended to be recreational and moderate.

Some "normal" trained athletes (without HCM) have hypertrophy of the left ventricle (i.e., thickening of the wall) resulting from intense and prolonged athletic training … which may resemble HCM. This distinction between the two diagnoses may be difficult to make in some athletes, but often can be resolved with non-invasive testing (i.e., echocardiography, MRI, and, in some cases, genetic testing). It is obviously an important distinction since HCM is a disease with potentially adverse consequences, while changes in heart structure produced only by athletic training (known as "athlete's heart") are not believed to represent a true pathologic abnormality or have important clinical implications to patients.

Treatments for HCM

There are several forms of treatment available directed toward improving heart function, relieving symptoms and preventing complications in HCM patients. Those with no symptoms generally do not require treatment, unless they are judged to be at high risk for sudden death. For patients who do require therapy for their disease, one or more of the following strategies may be considered.

Medical management

Medications are usually the first line of treatment for HCM patients experiencing heart failure symptoms of shortness of breath and chest pain associated with exertion, and many patients benefit from the administration of such medications with a reduction in those symptoms. A relatively small number of drugs are currently used in treating HCM, and the choice of which one to use first is often made on an individual patient basis. When children with HCM develop such symptoms they are treated with the same drugs, but in reduced dosage. The drugs most commonly used in HCM are described below.

Beta-blockers are a popular cardiovascular medication. There are approximately 20 different beta-blocking drugs available world-wide. Beta-blockers slow the heart rate, reduce the force of contraction, probably improve filling of the ventricles in diastole, decrease the oxygen demand of the heart, and may also decrease the degree of obstruction provoked during exercise. Beta-blockers are also widely used in medical practice for the treatment of other types of heart disease, including high blood pressure and heart failure following a heart attack, or other cardiomyopathies. However, sometimes beta-blockers can produce excessive fatigue, lightheadedness, nightmares, and occasionally impotence. But all these side effects are reversible once the drug is withdrawn. Several beta-blockers are available for use in HCM: propranolol (Inderal®), atenolol (Tenormin®), nadolol (Corgard®), and metoprolol (Lopressor®; Toprol XL®). Long-acting preparations of these drugs, requiring only a single daily dosage are now used predominantly. Termination of beta-blockers should be done by reducing the dose of the drug gradually over about a week. It is not advisable to suddenly stop taking a beta-blocker because of the chance your shortness of breath and/or chest pain may come back suddenly. Always consult your cardiologist prior to discontinuing any of these medications.

Calcium channel blockers. The second major group of drugs is calcium channel blockers, with verapamil (Calan®; Isoptin®) most commonly administered to HCM patients. This drug appears to relax the heart and improve filling of the ventricles (during diastole). Also, like beta-blockers, verapamil can cause slowing of the heart rate and lower blood pressure; some patients also experience constipation, dizziness, or ankle edema. However, other calcium antagonists such as nifedipine (Procardia-XL®) should be avoided because of the risk of inducing outflow obstruction. Beta-blockers and verapamil are usually not administered together because this combination may lower heart rate and/or blood pressure excessively. Another calcium blocker, diltiazem (Cardizem®; Dilacore-XL®), has also been used occasionally in HCM, but there are no data on its efficacy.

Disopyramide (Norpace®). This is a drug which relaxes the heart and is also an antiarrhythmic agent. Disopyramide has been used less commonly than beta-blockers and verapamil to treat HCM patients with symptoms. Nevertheless, disopyramide (which is usually administered with a beta-blocker) is unique among HCM drugs, with the capability to decrease obstruction at rest. Importantly, disopyramide apparently has little propensity to provoke arrhythmias in HCM.

Amiodarone. Amiodarone (Cordarone®; Pacerone®) is the most commonly used antiarrhythmic drug in HCM, usually to reduce the chances of recurrent episodes of atrial fibrillation. However, amiodarone does have several potential important side effects, especially sensitivity to the sunlight (which can be avoided with use of high SPF barrier creams and long-sleeved clothing), reversible effects on the thyroid gland, and occasionally damage to the lungs or liver. Periodically (every 6 months or so) monitoring of the liver, thyroid, and liver function should be preformed when a patient is taking amiodarone. For these reasons, it is always uncertain whether amiodarone can be tolerated for particularly long periods of time in any individual patient, particularly young people at high risk for sudden death. This is one of the reasons amiodarone has been abandoned as a primary treatment for high-risk HCM patients who may be susceptible to ventricular tachycardia and fibrillation and sudden death. Some cardiologists have used the antiarrhythmic drug *sotolol* (Betapace®) which combines some of the properties of amiodarone and a beta-blocker, but there are virtually no data in HCM patients. Other antiarrhythmic drugs such as quinidine and procainamide have been abandoned due to their propensity to induce important arrhythmias.

Diuretics. Most patients with HCM do not require diuretics (water tablets) for management of their symptoms. However, some severely symptomatic patients develop fluid retention, and in that situation diuretics, which increase urine flow, may be administered. The most common diuretics are furosemide (Lasix®), hydrochorothiazide (known as HCTZ), and a combination of hydrochlorothiazide and triamterene (Dyazide®, Maxzide®). Even though diuretics often eliminate fluid build-up in the lungs and in the extremities these drugs should be taken with caution in HCM patients for two reasons. First of all, dehydration may result, which could lead to an increase in obstruction and symptoms. Secondly, diuretics tend to cause electrolyte (potassium, magnesium, calcium) depletion, and that may predispose to dangerous arrhythmias. Therefore, patients who take diuretics are often checked by their physician for electrolyte deficiency (such as potassium) and are prescribed electrolyte supplementation in tablet forms.

Anticoagulants. Most patients with episodic or persistent atrial fibrillation should take anticoagulants ("blood thinners"; usually Coumadin®; warfarin) to prevent stroke, which may result if a clot forms due to stasis of blood in the atria, and a portion breaks off and travels through the arterial bloodstream to the brain. Such treatment requires monitoring with a blood test (called INR), approximately on a monthly basis. Given the potential complications of anticoagulation (e.g., hemorrhage from trauma), the decision of whether to begin anticoagulation may be a difficult one and obviously should be made in close consultation with your cardiologist. In some cases, standard aspirin is used as an anticoagulant. However, the effectiveness of Coumadin® and aspirin is not equal and the choice often depends on the degree of protection needed in a specific situation. There are no data on the efficacy of clopidogrel (Plavix®) in HCM.

Conversely, there are some drugs which should generally to be avoided in HCM. For example, medications which dilate peripheral vessels such as nitroglycerin and angiotensin-converting enzyme (ACE) inhibitors (lisinopril, ramipril) and angiotensin-receptor blockers (losartan and others) are not usually prescribed to patients with HCM because of their ability to cause an increase in obstruction.

Antibiotics. Although ***endocarditis*** is rare, patients with HCM and obstruction either at rest or with exercise, in which there is turbulent blood flow in the left ventricular outflow tract, should receive ***antibiotic prophylaxis*** prior to any dental procedures (including cleaning), as well as other surgical interventions. The American Heart Association's recommendations for bacterial endocarditis prevention appear in Table 2. Arrangements for antibiotic

Table 2 American Heart Association recommendations for antibiotic prophylaxis to prevent endocarditis (valve infection).

Dental procedures for which prophylaxis is recommended
- Dental extractions
- Periodontal procedures including surgery, scaling, and root planning, probing, and recall maintenance
- Endodontic (root canal) instrumentation or surgery only beyond the apex
- Subgingival placement of antibiotic fibers or strips
- Initial placement of orthodontic bands but not brackets
- Intraligamentary local anesthetic injections
- Prophylactic cleaning of teeth or implants where bleeding is anticipated

Other procedures for which endocarditis prophylaxis is recommended
- Respiratory tract
  - Tonsillectomy and/or adenoidectomy
  - Surgical operations that involve respiratory mucosa
  - Bronchoscopy with a rigid bronchoscope
- Gastrointestinal tract
  - Sclerotherapy for esophageal varices
  - Esophageal stricture dilation
  - Endoscopic retrograde cholangiography with biliary obstruction
  - Biliary tract surgery
  - Surgical operations that involve intestinal mucosa
- Genitourinary tract
  - Prostatic surgery
  - Cystoscopy
  - Urethral dilation

(continued)

Table 2 (*continued*).

Prophylaxis regimens for dental, oral, respiratory tract, or esophageal procedures (total children's dose should not exceed adult dose)

I Standard
  – Amoxicillin: Adults, 2.0 g (children, 50 mg/kg) given orally 1 hour before procedure.
II Unable to take oral medications
  – Ampicillin: Adults, 2.0 g (children 50 mg/kg) given IM or IV within 30 minutes before procedure.
III Amoxicillin/ampicillin/penicillin-allergic patients
  – Clindamycin: Adults, 600 mg (children 20 mg/kg) given orally 1 hour before procedure. *OR*
  – Cephalexin or cefadroxil: Adults, 2.0 g (children 50 mg/kg) orally 1 hour before procedure. *OR*
  – Azithromycin or clarithromycin: Adults, 500 mg (children 15 mg/kg) orally 1 hour before procedure.
IV Amoxicillin/ampicillin/penicillin-allergic patients unable to take oral medications
  – Clinidamycin: Adults, 600 mg (children 20 mg/kg) IV within 30 minutes before procedure. *OR*
  – Cefazolin: Adults, 1.0 g (children 25 mg/kg) IM or IV within 30 minutes before procedure.

Adapted from *Prevention of Bacterial Endocarditis: Recommendations by the American Heart Association* by the Committee on Rheumatic Fever, Endocarditis, and Kawasaki Disease. J Am Med Assoc 1997;277:1794–1801 and Circulation 1997;96:358–366. Reproduced with permission.

prophylaxis should be made directly with your dentist (or surgeon) at the time the appointment is made, well in advance of the procedure.

Implantable defibrillators

Those HCM patients clearly at high risk for sudden death may be candidates for an **implantable cardioverter-defibrillator (ICD)**, a sophisticated device which is permanently implanted internally and is capable of sensing potentially lethal arrhythmias and then automatically introducing a shock to terminate these arrhythmias and restore normal heart rhythm (Figure 24). At the same time, an ECG recording is generated directly by the device to precisely document the event. Recently, there has been much more experience with, and interest in, employing the ICD therapy in high-risk HCM patients with genetic heart diseases (such as HCM), including in some children. The ICD represents a major innovation, as it is capable of favorably changing the clinical course of HCM for many patients by preventing sudden death. In the largest study published to date (Figure 25), the ICD appropriately intervened, aborting potentially lethal arrhythmias in individual high-risk patients at a rate of 5% per year (>40% in 10 years, if extrapolated over time). This rate of discharge was highest if the ICD was placed because of a prior cardiac arrest (11% per year), but was also substantial in those patients for whom the device

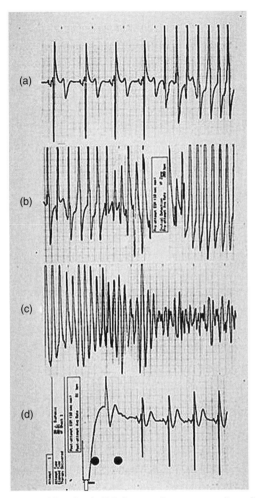

Figure 24 *ICD aborting sudden death*. This is a continuous recording of an electrocardio-gram obtained from the recording system of the ICD at the time of a life-saving event in a 36-year-old man with HCM. This patient, who had not previously experienced symptoms, received his ICD prophylactically because of high-risk status: he had extreme left ventricu-lar wall thickening and his younger brother had recently died suddenly of HCM. For almost 5 years, nothing adverse occurred. Then, early one morning while he was asleep at 1 a.m., normal heart rhythm converted suddenly to a life-threatening rhythm disturbance known as ventricular tachycardia (a). (b) Ventricular tachycardia continues and this is sensed by the device (as noted by the box). (c) While the device is charging (for 8 seconds), the situa-tion deteriorates with ventricular tachycardia converting to a particularly serious rhythm known as ventricular fibrillation in which the ventricles (two lower chambers) fibrillate and do not contract effectively to sustain a measurable blood pressure. (d) The ICD automati-cally delivers a shock (denoted by the arrow and box at lower left), which immediately con-verts the patient to a normal heart rhythm. Other than being awakened abruptly by the shock, the patient has experienced no difficulties during the ensuing 8 years.

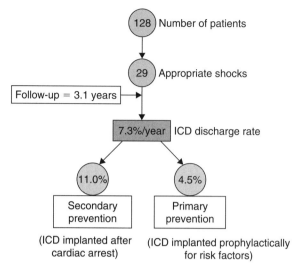

Figure 25 Outcome after ICDs were implanted in a large group of high-risk patients with HCM over a 3-year period. Extended data in 505 HCM patients are now available, and are very similar to these, but not yet published.

was implanted for one or more of the HCM risk factors … and without a prior major clinical event (about 4% per year). Most of those patients for whom the ICD is life saving are young and without significant symptoms.

Also, over the last few years, ICDs have become smaller and much easier to implant in unobtrusive positions on the chest, requiring in most instances only an overnight hospital stay without major surgery (Figure 26). The generator (containing the battery) is now, on average, 2½ × 2 inches and less than ½ inch thick, and fits just below the clavicle. ICD leads are now introduced into the heart chamber through the veins, avoiding major surgery.

Patients must also be aware of the possible complications associated with ICDs such as false-shocks due to fast but benign heart rates (in about 30% of patients, at present). Furthermore, there is a small chance of infection, and problems with the leads (usually breaking) are not uncommon and may occasionally require removal.

As the risk period in HCM is characteristically very long (theoretically 20–50 years in some patients), the ICD is likely to be a life-long treatment, thereby creating the crucial necessity for careful and consistent maintenance and interrogation of the device (usually 3–4 times per year), as well as regular battery replacement (currently at about 5-year intervals). We have knowledge of several HCM patients in whom the ICD discharged appropriately for the first time as long as almost 10 years after it was first implanted, as well as other patients who have survived for 25 or more

(a)

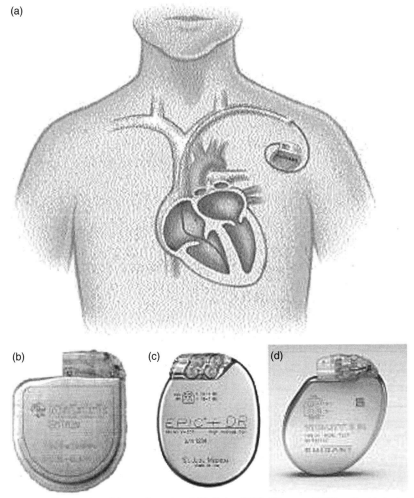

(b) (c) (d)

Figure 26 *The implantable cardioverter-defibrillator (ICD).* When an HCM patient is judged to be at high-risk this device can be permanently implanted to automatically detect and terminate life-threatening arrhythmias. (a) A small box measuring about 2 × 2½ inches is placed under the skin just below the clavicle (collar bone), and is attached to wires (called leads) introduced into the heart which are responsible for sensing (and recording) the heart rhythm … and delivering a defibrillation shock, if necessary, which restores normal electrical activity. (Bottom) Examples of ICD generators. (b) Courtesy of Medtronic Inc. (c) Courtesy of St. Jude Medical, Inc. (a and d) Courtesy of Guidant Corp.

years after cardiac arrest (without recurrence or ICD shock). These observations emphasize the unpredictable timing of these potentially lethal events and also the distinct possibility that they may occur only occasionally over a life-time.

In the future, we expect that ICDs will be offered as life-saving protection to many more HCM patients, certainly after they have already survived a cardiac arrest, but also prophylactically because of high-risk status (with one or more of the aforementioned risk factors) that is, *before* any major problems arise. However, it is important to note that the ICD is not a treatment for all HCM patients … only for those who are judged by their cardiologist to be truly at high risk. Furthermore, it should be emphasized that most HCM patients without currently known risk factors are at low (or possibly no) risk for sudden death. In high-risk patients there no longer appears to be a primary role for antiarrhythmic drugs (such as amiodarone) as primary alternatives to the ICD. These medications have not been proven to abolish the risk for sudden death, and also are likely to create important side effects requiring premature discontinuation of the drug over the long time periods which are usually necessary for administration to offer protection against sudden and unexpected death in HCM. However, your electrophysiologist may elect to use amiodarone (or other cardioactive drugs, such as beta-blockers) after defibrillator implantation principally to suppress heart rate and avoid inappropriate shocks during exercise.

Surgery

Surgery (the **ventricular septal myectomy** operation) is reserved for those patients with marked outflow obstruction who have severe symptoms uncontrolled by treatment with medications (Figure 27). The usual level of obstruction necessary to recommend surgery is a gradient of at least 50 mmHg either at rest or with exercise. With septal myectomy, the operating surgeon removes a small portion of the thickened muscle from the upper portion of ventricular septum, thereby widening the left ventricular cavity in that region, making it unlikely that the mitral valve will contact the septum in systole … and thereby relieving the obstruction. Some surgeons perform what is known as "extended" myectomy which removes tissue deeper into the ventricle (Figure 27). Relief of obstruction by myectomy is virtually always permanent.

Surgery for HCM should be performed only by surgeons familiar and experienced with this particular operation (usually at referral centers). This has created a situation where HCM patients requiring surgery have frequently traveled outside of their home communities for treatment. In experienced centers, operative mortality is now very low (1% or less), with most patients reporting long-lasting and significant improvement, or often abolition of symptoms. It is also now known that, by following large numbers of patients for many years after myectomy, the survival achieved is the same as that for the general population, and also better than for HCM patients with

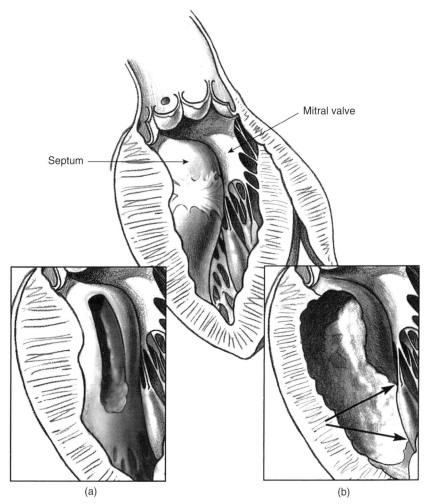

(a)   (b)

Figure 27 Diagram showing two operative approaches for performing septal myectomy in obstructive HCM. Typical outflow tract structure with hypertrophy of upper septum and obstruction due to systolic anterior motion of the mitral valve (center panel). (a) A standard rectangular myectomy is created from below the aortic valve to a point just beyond the point of obstruction, allowing for relief of the outflow gradient. (b) A much more substantial myectomy is performed by combining the standard operation with an extended muscle resection deeper into the septum. The portion of the myectomy trough toward the apex of left ventricle is much wider (arrows).

obstruction who do not undergo myectomy or any other major intervention (Figures 28 and 29). Surgery can be (and has been) performed safely and effectively in both children and in elderly patients with HCM. Operative risk for HCM appears to increase only when additional heart surgery (such as coronary artery bypass grafting) must also be performed at the same time.

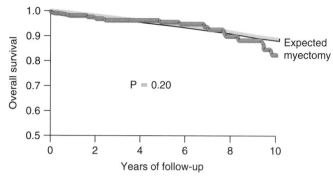

Figure 28 Survival of HCM patients many years after myectomy compared to survival of an age and gender matched general U.S. population (i.e., expected survival). There is no difference between the two curves and therefore myectomy can be considered as a treatment for restoring a patient's expected longevity.

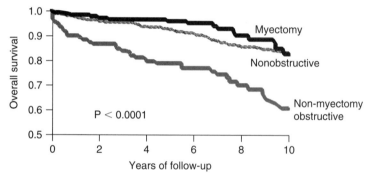

Figure 29 Survival, free from HCM-related death, comparing patients after myectomy with patients with HCM and obstruction who (for a variety of reasons) did not undergo myectomy, and HCM patients without obstruction who did not qualify for surgery based on customary practice criteria. Survival with myectomy is significantly superior to the other groups, particularly those patients with obstruction but without myectomy.

If the myectomy operation is performed properly, obstruction will be virtually obliterated under resting conditions and will not return. Therefore, heart failure due to obstruction is a reversible condition when treated with myectomy. Myectomy should only be performed by surgeons fully experienced with this operation. Patients should keep this important point in mind at which time they are being considered as a candidate for surgical intervention. Occasionally, in selected patients under special circumstances, instead of a myectomy operation, the surgeon may choose to replace the mitral valve with an artificial (usually mechanical) valve to relieve obstruction and symptoms. In some rare cases, mitral valve repair (instead of replacement) may accompany a myectomy.

Of course, some patients who meet the clinical criteria for surgery are not, in fact, optimal candidates for operation – either because of other complicating diseases, geographic inaccessibility to an experienced surgeon, particularly advanced age, and fear or lack of motivation for surgery.

Alcohol septal ablation (non-surgical myectomy)

A relatively new procedure for symptomatic patients with outflow obstruction has been devised to reduce the thickening of the upper septum (and thereby relieve outflow obstruction), without the need for open-heart surgery. Indeed, alcohol septal ablation appears to reduce obstruction and symptoms to a similar degree as surgery.

This technique involves injecting a small amount of absolute alcohol (about 2 ml) into a minor (small) branch of the left coronary artery that supplies the top portion of the ventricular septum, thus destroying heart cells and ultimately thinning that portion of the wall – and, in effect, intentionally producing a myocardial infarction and healed scar (i.e., a "heart attack"). The cavity of the left ventricle is thereby widened, permitting easier and more effective emptying of blood into the aorta – similar to the effects of myectomy. This technique is performed as part of a cardiac catheterization under local anesthesia. Although in a relatively early stage of development (compared to surgery), alcohol ablation represents a useful addition to the management options available to some selected HCM patients with severe drug-refractory HCM symptoms.

However, there are some important points concerning alcohol ablation to consider. The overall procedural mortality for the ablation procedure appears to exceed that for myectomy surgery in experienced centers. At present, the application of alcohol septal ablation to HCM patients remains a somewhat controversial and largely unresolved issue. Some interventional cardiologists advocate it with great enthusiasm, while other cardiologists (including virtually all HCM experts) suggest much more restraint until longer-term consequences of the procedure can be assessed more completely. Indeed, there is concern that ablations are being performed with increasing frequency by cardiologists new to this technique, and possibly in some patients with fewer symptoms than usually required for the traditional surgical candidate. *The HCMA believes that alcohol ablation is being recommended and used prematurely and excessively by some cardiologists and caution is advised in this regard.*

Therefore, most HCM experts, including those institutions endorsing this book, consider surgical myectomy to be the primary "gold standard" intervention for patients with unresponsive severe symptoms and obstruction ... and disability unresponsive to medication. HCM experts regard alcohol septal ablation as an acceptable treatment option only in certain selected HCM patients. These include patients who are elderly, with associated medical conditions that increase the risks of surgery, lack sufficient motivation, or have a strong preference against undergoing heart surgery. Therefore, alcohol ablation is intended to be a potential *alternative to surgery.*

Of note, alcohol septal ablation leaves patients with a heart scar which theoretically predisposes to important arrhythmias later in life (unlike surgical myectomy, which leaves no such scar). This risk has not yet been well documented, but the occurrence of serious arrhythmias is so unpredictable over long periods of time in young and middle-aged patients with HCM, that this possibility must be taken seriously. For this reason, we do not recommend septal ablation to young or even middle-aged adult patients at this time (and certainly not children); patients of advanced age (i.e., >65 years) may be more acceptable candidates.

Indeed, HCM referral institutions perform alcohol septal ablation only in operative candidates who otherwise are not optimal subjects for myectomy. In such environments, alcohol ablation is not regarded as either a cure or a primary treatment for this disease ... but rather a potentially useful addition to the available treatment strategies for selected patients with obstruction and severe symptoms. Also, the anatomy of the left ventricle and mitral valve, precise location of the obstruction within the chamber, and the size and distribution of the small coronary arteries used in the alcohol ablation procedure may vary considerably among patients – making some less optimal candidates for the ablation and more likely to benefit from surgery.

Pacemakers

Pacemakers are used in HCM for several reasons. Occasionally, when the normal electrical signal fails to traverse the ventricles, either because of sinus node failure or heart block, implanting a pacemaker is appropriate and necessary. This involves placing a small box containing a battery in the chest under the skin and passing fine wires through the veins to the heart in order to deliver the necessary signals so that the heart is automatically paced.

In the 1990s, many severely symptomatic patients with HCM and obstruction received dual-chamber pacemakers for the purpose of relieving symptoms and outflow obstruction, as a treatment alternative to the septal myectomy operation. However, much of the symptom improvement perceived by most patients was shown to be a **placebo effect**, rather than real change in the disease state, and the reduction in gradient was shown to be modest. Older patients with HCM (>65 years of age) have shown the most convincing positive effects from pacing. It is essential to keep in mind that the most important issue in the treatment of any patient with HCM is whether an intervention (including pacing) improves symptoms and quality of life, and not its precise effect on the degree of obstruction. Adult patients with coronary artery disease and/or severe heart failure are often treated with pacing (from both ventricles) – known as biventricular pacing. However, to date, this approach has rarely been used in HCM.

Heart transplantation and end-stage HCM

For a very small minority of HCM patients, heart transplantation may be recommended when there is severe, progressive disability and uncontrolled symptoms of shortness of breath with exertion, associated with marked impairment in the pumping action of the ventricles … and often accompanied by enlargement of the heart chambers and thinning of the left ventricular wall. This part of HCM often has the unfortunate label as the "end stage" (or sometimes the "dilated" or "burned-out" phase), and is the most common indication for heart transplantation within the disease spectrum of HCM. The "end stage" is ultimately uncommon, affecting only about 2–3% of patients. In this phase of the disease, spontaneously and without a triggering clinical event, the heart undergoes anatomic and functional changes due primarily to widespread ischemia and scarring of heart muscle. This process results in a form of heart failure more reminiscent of other diseases with greatly enlarged chambers (such as the dilated form of cardiomyopathy). As a result, the medical treatment for the end stage prior to heart transplantation will differ considerably from that typically employed in HCM, and include administration of beta-blockers (metoprolol, carvedilol) ACE-inhibitors (lisinopril, ramipril) or angiotensin-receptor blockers (losartan, valsartan, and others) and diuretics. Cardiologists may also choose to prescribe digoxin, spironolactone, and start an anticoagulant.

When the end stage is identified, it is often advised to contact a transplantation program and obtain their perspective on the requirements of being "listed" for heart transplant. The primary reason for this advice is that sometimes, after being stable for many years, patient's symptoms in the end-stage phase can progress rapidly and unpredictably. The process of evaluation for heart transplantation can take several months, and can be a daunting task for severely symptomatic, disabled patients. After transplantation, patients have a restored quality of life and in almost all cases can go back to their daily routine and jobs – and feel as good as they did before the end-stage process started. However, this "new lease on life" comes at the price of taking immunosuppressive drugs to prevent rejection of the transplanted heart, and compliance with post-transplantation medical appointments.

Of note, the "end-stage" phase represents an instance in the natural history of HCM, during which there is often considerable decrease in the thickness of the left ventricular wall, associated with an unfavorable clinical course. Therefore, the goal of "curing" HCM by reducing wall thickness (as has been proposed periodically for other patients) does not appear to be a realistic or achievable aspiration for the treatment of this disease.

It is evident from this discussion that HCM is a particularly heterogeneous disease, and certainly that concept applies directly to the selection of treatment options. The disease and treatment spectrum of HCM are summarized in Figure 30.

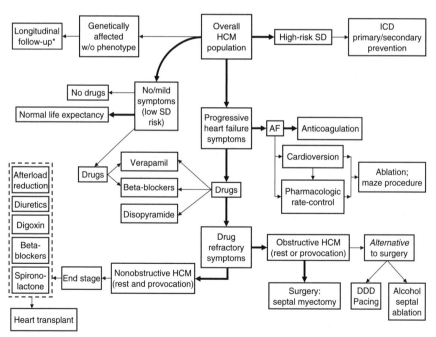

Figure 30 *Summary of treatment strategies for the very broad overall HCM disease spectrum.* AF = atrial fibrillation; ICD = implantable cardioverter-defibrillator.

Is a cure available?

HCM is a chronic disease

Patients often ask whether there is a known cure for HCM. Strictly speaking, a cure for this disease is not available … that is, if "cure" means the complete and absolute elimination of the entire disease process and all of its consequences. Therefore, HCM must be regarded, at present, as a chronic disease. However, it is also very important to emphasize that HCM is not only compatible with normal longevity (not uncommonly with little or no disability and without the need for major treatment interventions), but the more serious disease complications can often be managed and controlled with drugs or implantable devices.

Therefore, HCM does not necessarily shorten life or impact substantially on the quality of life. For example, in patients judged to be high risk for sudden death, an ICD will likely be protective from such an event. For that individual patient, there may be no other risks related to HCM and therefore the ICD could possibly be regarded selectively as an HCM "cure," i.e., allowing that particular patient to achieve normal or near-normal longevity.

Life with HCM: the long term

Patients with HCM often live with the fear that their life is destined to be short based solely on the diagnosis of HCM … and this is not correct. While HCM can be life threatening, it is also be compatible with a normal life span. This paradox is often the cause for confusion, frustration, and denial for many patients. At HCMA, we have many members who are enjoying long, meaningful, and relatively healthy lives. With the advances in our understanding of HCM and with early diagnosis and treatment, it is reasonable to expect that life spans will continue to be as long if not longer than in past generations for those with this complex disease. A life with minimal or no significant medical intervention is not only possible, but common for those with HCM.

Gene therapy

It is unlikely that, in the foreseeable future, gene therapy will be a workable or practical treatment approach for HCM. Reducing wall thickening and hypertrophy (i.e., normalizing the heart structure) by such means is not a reasonable aspiration for HCM patients and, in fact, has never been shown to be possible. Patients often inquire about the possibility of an HCM cure through gene therapy (in which "bad" genes are replaced by "good" or "normal" genes delivered directly into the body by a variety of methods), given the visibility of gene therapy and the human genome project provided by the news media. However, conceptually, gene therapy will be a very difficult process in a disease genetically transmitted as a dominant trait (such as is HCM). Standard models for which gene therapy has been proposed are other types of genetic diseases known as **recessive**. Also, gene therapy does not seem practical or largely applicable to HCM since the notion of introducing enough "good gene" to make all cells normal is regarded by molecular scientists as particularly daunting. Furthermore, such a treatment would not be without risk to patients, raising ethical issues as to which patients could (or should) be treated in this way. Keep in mind that even many patients with HCM experience a relatively benign course, and can even achieve normal life expectancy, without such heroic interventions. Therefore, in purely theoretical terms, gene therapy would necessarily have limited application and be confined to particularly high-risk patients and families, and even then probably in very young patients in whom hypertrophy had not yet become fully established. It is evident that, even if technically feasible, the selection of HCM patients for gene therapy could be as complex as the treatment itself.

Therapy for cardiovascular and other diseases with stem cells is currently an area of intense interest and study. However, stem cell therapy would not appear to be applicable to HCM since adding heart cells to a disease state in which the heart is already excessively thickened would not seem to be advisable.

Family screening

The majority of patients with HCM have at least one other affected relative (i.e., usually a parent, sibling, or child). When an individual is diagnosed with HCM all close relatives should be advised and afforded the option of screening for the disease with an echocardiogram and ECG. It is important to remember that such a family evaluation is potentially important because HCM may be present, even without associated heart symptoms. A standard non-invasive outpatient screening evaluation includes a personal and family history, physical examination, ECG, and echocardiogram.

The standard and principal diagnostic test for the clinical diagnosis of HCM is the two-dimensional echocardiogram (with Doppler). Hence, family screening for HCM is best carried out as it has been for many years – with the two-dimensional echocardiogram (and ECG). The purpose of screening is to identify what is known as the *phenotype* or overt expression of HCM – that is, the thickening of the left ventricular wall. In this regard, it is important to keep in mind an important distinction … while the mutant gene is present from birth, thickening of the left ventricular wall is delayed and almost always develops later (even decades later, in some cases). Sometimes HCM is referred to as a "congenital" heart disease (present from birth), but it is really only the genetic abnormality that is present from conception. This, of course, raises the unresolved question of when HCM becomes a "disease" – at birth, when the mutant gene is present, later when the heart wall becomes thick, or when symptoms occur. This particular nomenclature is often confusing to patients.

The heart wall thickening is most likely to be detected in the adolescent years. Wall thickness usually increases as children progress through puberty with accelerated body growth and maturation (approximately ages 12–17 years). Indeed, if a thickened wall becomes evident in an HCM family member on the echocardiogram during adolescence – and cannot be explained in any another way – it may be assumed to represent the mutant gene causing HCM. These changes in thickness with growth can be abrupt and striking and therefore the appearance of the heart can be altered substantially during the teenage years – from completely normal (or near-normal) thickness to a very thick left ventricle. HCM experts believe these changes in hypertrophy, while often alarming in appearance to the family (and even some physicians), nevertheless represent the expected ("normal") pattern in HCM (dictated by the DNA code), by which the heart reaches its mature structural form in this genetic disease. Therefore, the rapid growth of the heart, commonly seen in teenagers, does not, *per se*, represent clinical deterioration, or a warning of imminent danger. Also, the fear of many patients that their heart will continue to thicken throughout life, ultimately resulting in a catastrophic event, is completely unfounded. In fact, in the vast majority of patients, wall thickness does not increase measurably (and may even decrease slightly) with advancing age in adults (after approximately age 21 years).

Usually, if hypertrophy is not present on the echocardiogram by the time full growth and maturation is achieved (about age 17–19 years) then it is less likely for it to appear later in life. However, recent research has shown that this rule is not invariable and some family members may not first express their hypertrophy until mid-life or beyond. To date, only a very few genetically affected individuals have been known to develop hypertrophy for the first time after age 30 years, and certainly the frequency with which this occurs is unknown. Consequently, if a relative in an HCM family is "echo-negative" (and with a normal ECG) by the time adulthood begins, then there is a high likelihood (probably >95% or more) of not being affected by the mutant gene present in that family. Of course, if one family member has been successfully genotyped in the laboratory (i.e., the family HCM gene has been identified by genetic testing) then all the aforementioned uncertainty can be eliminated since it is relatively easy in such a circumstance to determine which other relatives are affected by the same mutation.

But, when should echocardiograms be performed routinely in children and other relatives within families with HCM? The current recommendations for screening are summarized in Table 3. Screening echocardiograms before the onset of puberty are largely optional since echocardiograms are rarely positive at that time, even in the presence of an HCM mutation, and recognition of the disease at this age usually does not necessitate treatment. An exception to this would be children in selected families with multiple occurrences of premature death due to HCM; in such a circumstance early identification of high-risk individuals would be advantageous by permitting measures for prevention of sudden death to be implemented. Early echocardiography is also recommended for those young family members who are in intense competitive athletic training programs, since HCM is the most important cause of sudden death during sports in young people

Table 3 Clinical screenings strategies with echocardiography (and ECG) for detection of HCM in families*.

<12 years old

Optional unless:
- Malignant family history of premature HCM death or other adverse complications
- Competitive athlete in an intense training program
- Onset of symptoms
- Other clinical suspicion of early left ventricular hypertrophy

12–21 years old[†]
- Every 12–18 months

>21 years old[†]
- Probably about every 5 years, or more at frequent intervals when there is a family history of late-onset HCM and/or malignant clinical course

---

From Maron et al. J Am Coll Cardiol 2004;44:2125–2132. Reproduced with permission.

*In the absence of laboratory-based genetic testing.

[†]Age range takes into consideration the acknowledged individual variability in achieving physical maturity.

and disqualification from that lifestyle would reduce risk. In general, we recommend serial echocardiograms (and ECGs) about every 12–18 months, from the onset of puberty (which may vary from about 10 to 13 years of age) throughout adolescence or, until the echocardiogram "converts" from normal to abnormal.

Because of the possibility of "late (adult) onset hypertrophy," into mid-life or even beyond, it is probably prudent for asymptomatic relatives with normal echocardiograms and ECGs at 18 years to obtain subsequent echocardiograms (and ECGs) at 5-year intervals to be sure that their hearts have not "converted" to HCM. This is admittedly a troublesome recommendation since "late-onset hypertrophy" is probably uncommon, and we know that 50% of those family members with extended screening would, in fact, be truly normal and free of an abnormal HCM gene. While it is certainly not our intention to introduce unnecessary anxiety to family members, (in the context of full disclosure) it is important that this information be conveyed as we know it at this time. This recommendation, of course, assumes that there has not been genetic testing to exclude an HCM mutation.

Strangely enough, the standard ECG may show an abnormal pattern in genetically affected children (or some adults) long *before* the echocardiogram changes from normal to abnormal and shows evidence of hypertrophy of the left ventricular wall. Therefore, the ECG can be the first clue or evidence of the HCM gene in young family members. In this way, the ECG can be a useful screening test for HCM in families, although it only records surface electrical signals and does not provide a direct image of heart structure (as does the echocardiogram).

Patients often ask whether the HCM gene can "skip" a generation. Rarely, adults in HCM families (with certain abnormal genes) may show no clinical evidence of HCM – that is, have a normal echocardiogram and ECG, and no symptoms, but nevertheless can pass the HCM gene onto the next generation. The gene does not really "skip" a generation, but rather it is expressed so subtlety so that we cannot see its representation on the echocardiogram. This is called *incomplete penetrance*.

Suggestions and helpful hints for screening examinations in children and teens:
• The day of the echocardiogram, explain to your child what the test is and what the room may look like:
  – The technician will take pictures of your heart.
  – The room will be a little dark to help the technician see your heart clearly on the screen.
  – There may be some strange sounds from the machine; this is from the Doppler and it is the machine magnifying the sounds of blood flow.

– There will be a gel applied to your chest and it may feel a little chilly or slimy.

– The doctor may come into the room to see how things are going.

• The day prior to the echocardiogram you may want to call the laboratory and determine whether they have a DVD or video machine available. If so, let your child bring their favorite movie or program with them.

• Bring age-appropriate distractions for the wait: MP3 players, books, puzzles, or stuffed animals.

• Bring a small snack and drink.

• Answer all the questions your child has; if you are unsure of the answer, call the doctor's office for more information, or ask others who have been through the process via the HCMA message board.

• As you experience several annual screenings with your child you may become skilled at noticing details on the echocardiogram. If you believe something has changed from a previous study … stay calm. Do not get emotional in front of your child, as that will unnecessarily cause anxiety. Remember, HCM is a treatable condition and is compatible with a normal life.

• After the examination, do something fun to allow you and your child to blow off some steam and relax. Go to a park, a favorite restaurant, a movie, or some other activity that you and your child enjoy doing together.

What about having children?: Pregnancy and delivery

Even if a child inherits the abnormal HCM gene, the degree to which he or she will be affected by the *disease* is largely unpredictable. There is no consistently reliable method for predicting precisely how severe HCM might be in an offspring and, in fact, there is considerable variability in this regard, even within individual families. A mildly affected parent can have a severely affected child, or vice versa. Alternatively, an entire family may have "benign" disease while other (albeit uncommon) families have "malignant" forms of HCM in which several relatives die prematurely or have severe disease and disability. Therefore, genetic counseling decisions to determine whether or not to have children must be an individual choice, based on many considerations, including the particular expression of HCM in the family.

For the vast majority of women with HCM, pregnancy and vaginal delivery poses no added risk and is well tolerated and safe. However, in the rare situation when a female HCM patient has severe symptoms or important arrhythmias, pregnancy could carry additional risk, and Caesarean section may be considered selectively to achieve some control over the medical circumstances. Obviously, such symptomatic pregnant women should have a cardiologist and access to specialized high-risk obstetrical care in order to make many important clinical decisions. Maternal death due to HCM as a consequence of childbirth is extraordinarily rare and virtually unreported.

However, women may find that they develop symptoms for the first time during pregnancy, or that preexisting symptoms are intensified. Issues related to taking cardiac drugs around the time of conception or during pregnancy arise in many cases. Drugs such as beta-blockers, calcium channel blockers (e.g., verapamil) taken by the mother have access to the fetus, because they are capable of crossing the placental barrier, and could in theory damage the baby. However, there is little direct evidence that the fetus can be damaged due to the administration of these drugs to the mother. Nevertheless, it is best to be cautious, if at all possible, and avoid all drugs during pregnancy (certainly in the first trimester). For all these reasons it is prudent for patients with HCM to plan their pregnancy in advance and discuss all pertinent medical issues at an early stage with their cardiologist and obstetrician. Also, it may be best to avoid, if possible, epidural anesthesia at delivery (particularly in women with obstruction), as this occasionally causes an excessive fall in blood pressure and therefore could increase obstruction.

Routine medical care

Patients with HCM should be seen regularly by a cardiologist near their home even if they are stable and do not develop new complaints. Clinic visits on an annual basis seem to work out best. Many patients complain that their cardiologist openly expresses inexperience with HCM. This, of course, is not an uncommon occurrence because of the relative infrequency of HCM in the general population and in cardiology practice. Some patients alleviate this frustration by electing to be evaluated and followed concurrently by an HCM consultant – that is, a cardiologist with special interest and expertise in HCM. Please contact the HCMA for names of HCM experts (Tel: 973 983 7429; Fax: 973 983 7870; e-mail: **support@4hcm.org**). Links to HCM specialty centers can be found on the HCMA website (**www.4HCM.org**). If you do not have Internet access, personally contact our office for HCM specialty center contact information. HCM patients should also maintain other aspects of their health and well-being such as annual examinations for non-cardiac-related problems. Of course, for those patients who are symptomatic and require treatment, more frequent follow-up may be required with a cardiologist as well as with another subspecialist such as an electrophysiologist (e.g., if a defibrillator is implanted). Generally, if the patient is stable and new issues do not arise, medical visits no more frequent than at 1-year intervals (with history and physical examination, echocardiogram, ECG, and ambulatory Holter ECG) is customary practice.

General lifestyle advice

Diet

Sensible eating habits are encouraged to maintain body weight within the normal range for height and age. If an individual is overweight, this places extra unnecessary strain on the HCM heart, as it would for any cardiac condition. Attention should also be paid to cholesterol levels, as would be advised for any patient. However, we wish to emphasize that elevated cholesterol is a risk factor for coronary artery disease, and not specifically for HCM. No special diet or vitamin supplementation is required for HCM. Of note, a rapid increase in weight is likely to be due to fluid retention and requires consultation with your doctor. Excessive salt intake should be avoided (unless specifically prescribed by your doctor), but unless heart failure is in its advanced stages, low salt diets are not usually advised.

Exercise

For most patients, HCM will not interfere importantly with lifestyle. Some individuals may have symptoms triggered by exertion and find that they cannot undertake as much physical work or recreation as other people their age. Under these circumstances, medical advice should be sought before undertaking physically demanding activities. Patients with HCM and symptoms such as shortness of breath, chest pain, or lightheadedness during activity (even if mild) should not extend themselves into physical activities that have the effect of provoking or accentuating symptoms. Such symptoms can be regarded as warning signs that heart function has been impaired. It is best to consider the axiom: have a good measure of respect for your disease (in this case HCM) and do not extend yourself beyond a reasonable threshold.

Most experts believe individuals with a confirmed diagnosis of HCM should not participate in most organized, competitive sports or other intense physical activities, as discussed in the section on Special consideration: Athletes and sports activities (golf and bowling are exceptions). This recommendation is based on the observation that intense physical exertion appears to predispose some susceptible individuals with HCM to arrhythmias and possibly sudden death.

Nevertheless, after these considerations are taken into account, it is a reasonable expectation that most affected individuals with HCM can adopt a normal or near-normal lifestyle, including many recreational physical activities, as long as they are undertaken in *moderation*. HCM patients should seek the advice of their cardiologist with regard to precisely what type of recreational exercise program should be implemented. In addition, American Heart Association recommendations are available to serve as a useful guide to these difficult decisions (Table 1).

Exercise programs for patients with HCM should not be confused with participation in competitive athletics or certain intense recreational sports. However, HCM patients are not compelled to lead a completely sedentary lifestyle. For example, walking and toning (without free weights) are two generally acceptable forms of exercise. However, all systematic exercise programs should be initiated with some caution.

In many families, sports have been traditional or play a very large role in daily life. These activities may have, in fact, become a major focus and important part of the social life of not only the child but the entire family. After a child has received a diagnosis of HCM it will be difficult for all parties (regardless of age) to understand that they can no longer participate in competitive sports. Indeed, when a diagnosis of HCM is made in a committed athlete it is perhaps more devastating in many ways than the same diagnosis in a non-athletic child. These children will require assistance to redirect their time and energy to other activities (that may include certain recreational sports), or in some cases to more acceptable competitive sports such as golf or bowling. Therefore, it is important to encourage the child to maintain existing relationships with friends in sports, but at the same time extend their network to individuals who participate in other activities.

At the same time it will also be difficult for parents who have developed social contacts associated with these sporting events, to no longer be able to participate. Some parents can find it just as difficult to deal with this loss as does the child. You may try to find alternative family activities in which new friends and traditions are developed to compensate, at least in part, for the feeling of loss.

Keep in mind that habitual, vigorous exercise has many benefits in middle-aged and older individuals for preventing the adverse consequences of coronary artery disease … but this is a much different situation than in HCM. It is neither possible nor advisable to view athletic training as a form of treatment for HCM. In particular, patients with symptoms of HCM, such as shortness of breath or chest pain, should not try to mitigate those symptoms by "exercising through" such complaints.

Alcohol

Patients with HCM should avoid excessive consumption of alcohol because of its potentially adverse effects on heart muscle and vasculature, specifically a decline in the pumping capacity of the heart and a rise in blood pressure. One study has shown that outflow obstruction may actually increase after very small amounts of alcohol, probably due to dilation of peripheral blood vessels produced by the drug. On the other hand, modest consumption of beer or wine is certainly acceptable.

Viagra

Viagra® (sildenafil citrate) Levitra® (vardenafil) and Cialis® (tadalafil) are the drugs available for the treatment of erectile dysfunction for which sudden death and other adverse consequences have been reported in a small number of symptomatic patients with coronary artery disease. However, because it is a much less common disease, there are no specific data governing the side effects of these medications in HCM. Nevertheless, there are important theoretic reasons to avoid these drugs if you have HCM. Since sidenafil, vardenafil, and tadlafil dilate arterial and venous vessels they could increase obstruction and in this way be adverse to HCM patients. Therefore, we believe patients with HCM should avoid Viagra®, Levitra®, and Cialis® until more data are available.

Flu vaccination

"Flu shots" may be recommended by your doctor to prevent influenza, particularly in very young and elderly individuals. Having HCM does not exclude this treatment, although you should be aware that there are occasional side effects from the vaccine (which also may not provide absolute protection against infection).

Weight management and obesity in HCM

The medical literature contains many articles describing the adverse cardiovascular effects of obesity. There are an estimated 75 million Americans who are more than 30 pounds over their ideal body weight. Mayo Clinic data show that patients with HCM who have weight-related medical conditions such as diabetes, systemic hypertension, and coronary artery disease face greater complications and less favorable future when compared to those of average weight. Patients with HCM face additional challenges when dealing with long-term weight management issues. Many patients cannot exercise regularly and adopt a sedentary lifestyle out of necessity. Certainly, the combination of a sedentary existence and chronic disease such as HCM makes weight loss difficult. Furthermore, obesity can worsen heart-related symptoms and substantial uncertainty may arise regarding whether symptoms are due to HCM directly or at least in part due to the patient's weight gain. It is critical for such patients to work closely with cardiac professionals to create a strategy and workable physical activity program to reduce weight.

Emotionally, weight maintenance can be just as debilitating as HCM. Patients should not be too hard on themselves regarding their weight, but should take steps to improve their overall health. Taking small steps to make long-term changes in eating habits and exercise is the way to start. It is important to remember that you will not necessarily see huge changes over short periods of time … but if you stick with healthy habits, they will pay off with gradual weight loss over time.

Finally, the subject of weight loss to an obese patient can itself create stress, depression, and feelings of failure. However, it is important to directly face the issue to improve overall health and start on the road to weight reduction. This will likely be a trial-and-error process until you find the weight loss method that works best for you. However, fad diets, over the counter diet pills, and starvation diets are not the way to safely lose meaningful weight. Creating a healthy eating plan in coordination with an exercise program will lead to gradual weight loss which is more likely to result in real weight loss over time.

Other restrictions

Acute severe loss of blood or body fluid: hemorrhage, diarrhea, and vomiting, if excessive, can lead to unfavorable consequences such as increase in obstruction. Seek medical attention should you experience severe diarrhea or vomiting.

Prolonged standing in hot conditions or very hot baths or showers: may predispose to fainting or near-fainting.

Anesthesia: special attention is required to avoid a sudden drop in blood pressure. There have been a few reports suggesting an increased risk associated with epidural anesthesia during delivery; this procedure should probably be avoided in HCM patients, particularly in the presence of outflow obstruction.

Prolonged exposure to extreme environmental temperatures (hot or cold): can predispose to unfavorable consequences such as arrhythmias.

Adapting to HCM psychologically

The initial diagnosis of HCM, which often comes as a complete surprise, can actually have a profound psychological impact (Table 4). Furthermore, the effect of chronic illness (such as HCM) on a patient and family is similar to that of other emotional trauma, but with certain differences. Chronic diseases produce the feelings of fear, grief, and loss that are essentially unending. HCM (which often affects young people and conveys a risk for sudden cardiac death in some patients) presents patients and their families with a lack of predictability which itself may make adjustment to life more difficult. There is constant living with the unknown and an acute sense that any personal control over events is lacking. This circumstance may be perceived as "living with a sword over one's head." In contrast, in most other instances of loss, as terrible as they are, there is at least a finality that must be accepted; shock and denial give way to acceptance and adaptation.

Imagine the following scenario. Someone says to you: "Carry this beeper. One day it may go off and you must respond immediately and correctly. It will be the most important moment of your life. It could go off next week, next year, or 10 years from now … but be ready." This situation can create chronic anxiety and anger in patients, their family, and in friends as well … and this is essentially what happens with a disease such as HCM. A medical condition can itself become an anxiety state characterized by preoccupation and hyperalertness, and can paralyze the patient's adjustment to daily life activities. Eventually, depression can result when the constant state of readiness (and often a sense of hopelessness) gradually wears down the patient's reserves. There is often a profound sense of unfairness ("how and why did this happen to me"), but also the realization that life is imperfect. The trauma created by chronic diseases can also result in

Table 4 Checklist for the newly diagnosed with HCM.

---

1 Speak to your cardiologist about his/her experience level with HCM.

2 Ask your cardiologist his/her feelings on working in partnership with an HCM specialty center to manage your care.

3 Make sure all tests have been performed to ensure thorough risk stratification:
   (a) Echocardiogram
   (b) Electrocardiogram
   (c) Holtor monitor
   (d) Stress test/stress echo.

4 Discuss with your doctor your treatment options:
   (a) If medications are prescribed, make sure you are clear on the dosage, timing, and side effects you may encounter, and when to talk to your cardiologist.
   (b) If an ICD or pacemaker, is prescribed, make sure you consult with an electrophysiologist prior to implantation.
   (c) If surgery is recommended, make sure you ask how many procedures have been performed at the center and how often they are done. HCMA highly recommends only centers which regularly perform myectomies, and have many years of experience in this operation.
   (d) If you have been recommended for alcohol septal ablation (also known as PTSMA or TASH), we suggest a complete evaluation by an HCM specialty center and careful adherence to the ACC/ESC Consensus Document guidelines on the treatment of HCM.

5 Discuss your employment situation with your cardiologist and make sure you can safely perform the duties required. If you cannot perform at work, ask your physician to write a letter to your Human Resources Department with a request for an Americans with Disabilities Act Accommodation.

6 Notify your first-degree family members that they will need to have screening for HCM. The screening should include an ECG, echocardiogram, consultation with a cardiologist, and a plan for future screenings on an age-appropriate basis.

---

re-prioritization of life goals and values – which may represent a positive consequence of an otherwise negative situation.

Disruption of the family homeostasis and the roles that members have played for years can be thrown into disarray. There may also be substantial guilt involved in HCM families – that is, for having transmitted the gene and disease to children. This may also relate to the dilemma faced by many patients, of deciding to have children (and take the chance of transmitting the mutant gene).

"Genetic guilt," as we often refer to it at the HCMA, is a natural emotion on the part of a parent affected by HCM who has a child with HCM. However, if a parent feels "genetic guilt" over the genetic material that made his/her child's abnormal heart, they should also be prepared to take credit for the wonderful genetic contributions made to create that beautiful smile, loving eyes, adorable laugh, or wonderful sense of humor.

Therefore, genetic counseling is an important component of treatment for HCM, as it may help to answer difficult and delicate questions for patients. Certainly, in many families there is not an absolutely correct answer to questions about HCM, as a number of considerations may be involved, including the variable clinical expression of the gene defect within and between families. Most importantly, for the majority of patients with HCM it is not necessary to live in terror of the possibility of deterioration and premature death, since it is now evident that this disease often has a benign course consistent with normal life expectancy.

Chronic diseases such as HCM present a series of dilemmas and a continuum of choices for patients. As a goal, we recommend achieving a psychological state somewhere in between the following extremes:

• From ignoring your symptoms and "toughing it out" – to over-reacting to your symptoms.

• From keeping your illness a secret and risking deception – to talking too openly and risking the perception of self-pity.

• From asking for help and risking becoming a burden – to holding on to your independence and risking isolation.

• From insisting that your family and friends treat you as normal and denying them the expression and release of their feelings – to letting your family and friends protect you and risk becoming overly dependent or child-like.

• From pushing your body to its physical limits and risking self-harm – to playing it safe and becoming an invalid.

• From living in terror of degeneration and death and risking immobilization – to regarding each day as a special and pristine opportunity.

• From insisting on controlling your life at the risk of frustration – to going with the flow and risking passivity.

• From being angry at your circumstances and risking bitterness – to focusing only on your blessings and risking self-delusion.

Fortunately, it is characteristic of human beings that a capacity for strength can be drawn from adversity. This can be aided by mutual support between patients and their families and by interaction between patients afflicted by the same disease. This process includes acknowledging what could have been and accepting and adapting to the reality of the given situation ... and also finding ways to make your life meaningful despite a chronic illness. It is important that as many family members or extended family and friends as possible participate in this renewal. The family that has been traumatized by chronic illness (in this case, by HCM) can thereby take collective pride in a new-found strength.

Finally, patients should refrain from seeking miracle solutions and should be cautious and discriminating about accepting seemingly unrealistic, dramatic predictions about disease cures, regardless of the source. Perhaps, it is best to regard most treatment advances in HCM in the context of *controlling* the disease, rather than as *cures* which obliterate the disease.

Driving

There are two different standards that apply to driving in the United States: commercial and personal driving. A diagnosis of HCM should have no bearing on a patient's personal driving privileges and license. If syncope (fainting) or near-syncope (near-fainting) has been experienced, the physician may advise the patient not to drive until these symptoms can be better controlled and understood.

To obtain a commercial driver's license (CDL), there are specific fitness guidelines. These guidelines do change from time to time, and therefore you may want to consult the Department of Transportation website for the latest information (http://www.fmcsa.dot.gov).

Currently, the CDL standard that applies to HCM patients is found in the Cardiovascular Advisory Panel Guidelines for the Medical Examination of Commercial Motor Vehicle Divers, FMCSA-MCP-02-002 October 2002, which specifically states the following:

"Irrespective of symptoms, a person should not be certified as a commercial driver if a firm diagnosis of HCM is made on echocardiography."

However, there is also an appeal process, and with a favorable evaluation from a cardiologist, it may be possible to eventually obtain a commercial driver's license. Re-evaluation is required annually, and a repetitive appeal process may be necessary. Therefore, we do not advise careers in this field for patients with HCM.

If you cannot walk long distances without symptoms such as shortness of breath, chest pain, or lightheadedness it is suggested you apply for a handicapped parking permit. It is advised that patients who even occasionally have such symptoms request the handicapped parking permit as it is difficult to predict a "bad day" in advance. In many cases this only involves a simple form that can be obtained from your local motor vehicle office (but must be signed by your doctor).

If you have an implantable defibrillator, consult with your doctor regarding local regulations governing automobile driving with these devices. In several states it is suggested that defibrillator patients should not drive for up to 6 months after their implant. At this time there does not appear to be a law governing this, and it is simply a recommendation. You and your physician should discuss your individual situation and decide what is in your best interest.

Traveling

You need to think about your health before you plan a trip. Remember to bring all medications with you and it is always a good idea to keep a letter in your possession explaining your medical condition. In U.S. airports, you can ask for assistance to be transported to your gate; foreign airports vary greatly and you should ask your travel agent to make arrangements for you. For those who are more symptomatic, it is critical to remember the importance of pacing yourself while on vacation, or you may become fatigued and will not enjoy yourself. Call ahead to see how far away the attractions are that you wish to see, and if necessary arrange for a motorized scooter or wheelchair. For example, major theme parks provide rental scooters and wheelchairs on site. If you are on a business trip allow ample travel time to arrive and rest before your meeting.

Commercial airline travel itself (at the altitudes conventionally involved) poses no risk to HCM patients. Caution should be exercised in scheduling vacations or trips to remote destinations where the level of medical care is rudimentary and where specific knowledge of HCM may be virtually non-existent. The same considerations apply to traveling on cruise ships where the level of medical care may not be consistent and, in some instances, suboptimal for a patient with HCM. If you have an implantable defibrillator and are planning a trip you may want to contact your electrophysiologist (or the device manufacturer) to identify the nearest suitable hospital to your vacation/business destination.

Customer service:

Medtronic, Inc.	+1 800 328 2518
710 Medtronic Parkway	+1 763 514 4000
Minneapolis, MN 55432-5604, USA	www.medtronic.com
Guidant Corporation	+1 800 227 3422
4100 Hamline Avenue North	+1 651 582 4000
St. Paul, MN 55112-5798, USA	www.guidant.com
St. Jude Medical, Inc.	+1 800 328 9634
One Lillehei Plaza	+1 651 483 2000
St. Paul MN 55117-9913, USA	www.SJM.com

Military service

For those wishing to enter the Armed Forces. Careers in the military are not encouraged for those with HCM for a variety of reasons. However, if one wishes to pursue this career path you should be aware of the following. As a general guideline the military will disqualify any person with "hypertrophy" or "dilation" of the heart. If a person with HCM wishes to enter the military there is an appeal process in which a petition can be made to the Service Waive Authorities for re-evaluation. If a person has long-term disease stability a waiver may be awarded. However, due to the variable nature of HCM it is unlikely that such a waiver would be awarded. If HCM is knowingly misrepresented at recruitment or service entry, and is established later, that person will be removed from the military and possibly prosecuted.

For those currently serving in the military. Many factors are evaluated by the military in determining whether a person with any newly discovered medical condition may remain in active service. Several issues will be considered in the case of a new HCM diagnosis including (but not limited to) length of service, job assignment, and qualifications. If someone is early in their career it is unlikely that the military will retain that person, who may then wish to apply for military disability. Military disability will pay a portion of your wages, but is not equivalent to Social Security Disability. The intent of military disability is, in most cases, to return that person to civilian life where employment will be available.

If the person is to remain in the military (and may already have an extensive career) it is likely that an assessment of the specific job functions can be requested. If that person is "fit for duty" they may remain in their assignment. If not, a new position and revised training program may be provided. However, with increasing frequency, the military is attempting to ensure – for matters of public safety, but also in the best interests of soldiers with a disease such as HCM – that recruits are World Wide Qualified. This means that person must be able to work any place the military may send them, without consideration for the availability of specific or specialized medical treatment. For example, if a person has an ICD and is stationed in a remote area, would the military be able to provide the care necessary to ensure that person's health and well-being?

The Americans with Disabilities Act does not provide protection for those in the U.S. Military. If you live outside the United States you should check with your local military recruitment center to inquire as to the military guidelines in your country.

Social Security benefits

Those in the United States who have severe limitation in daily life functions because of HCM may be eligible for Social Security Disability Insurance (SSI) coverage. However, a diagnosis of HCM is not itself sufficient to claim disability under SSI. Social Security defines "disability" as the inability to do any kind of work for which you are suited and trained; your disability is expected to last for at least 1 year.

The definition of disability under Social Security is different than in other programs. Social Security pays only for total disability. No benefits are payable for partial or for short-term disability. Disability under Social Security is based on the inability to work. You are considered disabled under Social Security rules if you cannot perform work that you did before and Social Security decides that you cannot adjust to other employment because of your medical condition(s). Social Security program rules also assume that working families have access to other resources to provide support during periods of short-term disabilities, including workers' compensation, insurance, savings, and investments.

You may receive Social Security Disability benefits at any age. If you are receiving such benefits at age 65 years, that amount will become your retirement benefit. Your dependants may be eligible for additional Social Security insurance benefits if your household income is low enough to create financial need. They include:

• Your unmarried children, including step-children, adopted children or, in some cases, grandchildren, under the age of 18 years (or 19 years if still in a full-time high school student).

• Your unmarried child, 18 years or older, if your disability started before the age of 22 years.

• Your spouse if 62 years or older, or any age if he or she is caring for a child of yours who is under 16 years or disabled, and also receiving disability checks.

• Your disabled widow or widower 50 years or older. The disability must have occurred before your death or within 7 years after your death.

• Your disabled ex-wife or ex-husband who is 50 years or older, if the marriage lasted at least 10 years.

Your local Social Security office will send your application to the Disability Determination Service (DDS) office in your state. A team consisting of a physician (or psychologist) and a disability evaluation specialist will consider all facts and decide if you are "disabled" by their definition. They determine whether you can perform work-related activities such as walking, sitting, lifting, and carrying.

If your claim is denied there are four levels of appeal available. As this is a complicated process, many choose to have an attorney represent them. To secure a lawyer, contact your local Bar Association for the names of disability attorneys in your area. For more information on Social Security, call them directly at 800 772 1213.

Family and Medical Leave Act

The Family and Medical Leave Act (FMLA) became effective in 1993. The purpose of the Act is to help balance the demands of the workplace with the needs of families by allowing eligible employees to take up to 12 weeks of unpaid, job-protected leave (during any 12-month period) for specific family emergencies such as serious illness or the birth of a child. Employers who have 50 or more employees working 20 or more weeks in the current or preceding calendar year and who are engaged in commerce are covered as well as public agencies (including governmental agencies and schools). To be eligible an employee must work:

1 For a covered employer at least 12 months.
2 At least 1,250 hours during the past 12 months; and at a location where at least 50 other employees are living within 75 miles of the workplace.

Many states have their own version of FMLA that run in conjunction with the Federal program. For specific information about the FMLA in your state, check with the State Department of Labor.

Health insurance

Your choice of health insurance can have a dramatic effect on the level of health care you receive. In the United States most people are insured through employer-based programs in which individuals are given options to review on an annual basis. Plans vary in coverage and cost but looks can be deceiving. Health Maintenance Organizations (HMOs) are normally the least expensive in terms of premiums, but also have the most restrictions and are often difficult to navigate if you are living with an uncommon condition like HCM. HMOs often claim to have doctors within their network who can evaluate your HCM; however, these doctors are often general cardiologists with no specific expertise in HCM. In general, HMOs are not the best option for patients with HCM.

Preferred Provider Organizations (PPOs) allow for in-and-out of network care and normally have premiums that are reasonable. PPOs allow the patient to seek out care with the most experienced centers and, in most cases, the major HCM centers participate with many large health care carriers' plans, thus keeping patients "in network." However, in the event you fall "out of network" you would have to pay a deductible in order to receive care in an experienced center, unlike HMOs who can refuse to pay any portion of the claim.

Point of Service (POS) plans can be difficult to understand as some have "referral required" clauses which make them more like a disguised HMO. However, if the POS has no referral required it will, in most cases, act more like a PPO.

Traditional indemnity plans are making a come-back and are a very good option as they simply provide coverage on a percentage split, 80% paid by the insurance carrier and 20% by the patient up to an out-of-pocket maximum of a set amount. These plans allow for the greatest freedom and are priced rather competitively.

Patients may meet financial criteria for state subsidized health care, Medicaid, which will provide some coverage. In the event the patient is qualified for Social Security either based on age or disability they may qualify for Medicare, in which case purchasing a Medicare supplement is advised.

The Health Insurance Portability and Accountability Act of 1996 (HIPAA) set forth federal rules for preexisting medical conditions. Under HIPAA preexisting conditions must be covered by a new plan as long as the participant has maintained some form of coverage without a break of 63 days. This means you can leave one job and start a new one without the ability of the plan disqualifying coverage for your HCM treatment as long as you have not broken coverage for 63 days. You may need to purchase COBRA coverage to protect you in such circumstances.

Life insurance

While the diagnosis of HCM will not always leave you "uninsurable," it may nevertheless result in very high premiums. You must disclose all medical information to the insurance company. With this in mind, it may be a wise idea to purchase coverage *prior to* being screened for HCM. If you have already been diagnosed with HCM you can purchase coverage from a number of "assigned risk" carriers. A better idea is to maximize any group insurance your employer, credit card company, or civic organization may offer.

Coverage for children may be taken as a "rider" on an existing adult policy. These provisions are in most cases "non-medical," which means that no medical questions are asked regarding the child. Many such "riders" can be converted to a separate policy at age 18 years, and at as much as 5 times the original value. This is a good way to ensure coverage for the child into adulthood.

Special considerations for implantable defibrillators

Patients and their families may have numerous questions about the ICD and how it might change their lives, particularly since it is likely to be a chronic treatment (Table 5). Many of these questions should be answered by the electrophysiologist responsible for your device, since these issues may differ on a case-by-case basis, and should be tailored to your own clinical situation and activity level. Regarding questions about the potential interaction between the ICDs and *electromagnetic* fields in the environment,

Table 5 What to expect from a defibrillator implant (ICD).

- Normally, the device is implanted in your upper chest, slightly below your collarbone; you will have a scar about 2 inches long. The leads are introduced through a vein.
- The first implant creates more discomfort than a replacement because a "pocket" is created.
- Bring a button-down shirt to leave the hospital in, as you will not be able to lift your arm over your head for a few days to 2 weeks.
- The use of modern conscious sedation minimizes any discomfort to the patient and eliminates the need for general anesthesia.
- Your leads need time to set within your heart, so you will not be able to lift anything over 10 pounds for a few weeks. You should be able to drive in 1–2 weeks. Talk to your electrophysiologist about specific time frames for returning to work, driving, and lifting, as the time may vary depending on your personal situation.
- Watch for signs of infection when you get home from the hospital; should you start to run a fever, notify your doctor at once.
- If your device delivers a shock, and you are feeling satisfactory afterwards, let your doctor or nurse know. You can wait until normal business hours to contact them. However, if you receive multiple shocks, are feeling ill afterwards, or you still perceive your heart is racing or beating too slowly, you should call 9-1-1 (emergency).
- Let someone at work know about your device. In the event that your ICD shocks you while at work make sure a co-worker can help you get the care you may need.
- If a child, teen, or young adult is having a device implanted, you may want to talk to his/her friends and their parents to explain the ICD. Young people spend a great deal of time with friends, and it is important that they know what to do in the event of a shock and also that life with an ICD is not so unusual.
- You must have your ICD checked every few months, the average is 3–4 months, but this varies somewhat from center to center.
- ICDs are man-made items, thus subject to imperfection. This is very rare but it can occur. In the event your device is "recalled," do not panic. This does not necessarily mean that your ICD must be removed and replaced. For example, it may mean that programming has to be changed or that the device needs to be assessed for a specific problem.
- If your ICD "beeps," you should notify your electrophysiologist immediately.

---

it is important to first understand the nature of an electromagnetic field, which is an invisible line of force resulting from electricity use, such as devices plugged into an outlet or operated by a battery.

Most of the equipment and appliances patients come into contact with on a daily basis will not affect an ICD. However, it is generally a good idea for patients to keep their distance from devices that generate large amounts of electromagnetic interference such as industrial welding instruments, anti-theft systems frequently found in stores, and large electrical generators (such as power plants), diathermy, electrocautery, as well as magnetic resonance imaging devices. Nevertheless, ICD recipients should be able to safely operate most household appliances, tools, and machines that are properly grounded and in good repair. Some examples that cause no interference include:

- Microwave ovens
- Metal detectors
- Televisions, AM/FM radios, VCRs
- Tabletop appliances such as electric toasters, blenders, knives, and can-openers
- Hand-held items such as shavers and hair-dryers
- Electric blankets and heating pads
- Major appliances including washers, dryers, and electric stoves
- Personal computers, photocopiers, and electric typewriters
- Light industrial equipment such as drills and table-saws (*not* including battery-powered tools)
- Dental drills

Defibrillators are sensitive to particularly strong electrical or magnetic fields, which have the potential to deactivate some devices, although this occurs only on very rare occasions. In some cases an ICD device may emit a sound if it is too close to a magnet. If this happens, it is important to move away from the object and location immediately. The potential sources of strong electrical and magnetic fields listed below should be kept at least 12 inches (30 cm) away from an ICD pulse generator:

- Stereo speakers from large systems, transistor radios, "boom boxes," or similar instruments
- Possibly some digital cell phones
- Engines with alternators emitting magnetic fields
- Strong magnets
- Magnetic wands used by airport security, and in other circumstances
- Battery-powered cordless power tools such as screwdrivers and drills

Airport security alarm systems (both the portals through which a person walks or the hand-held wand) employ magnetic fields for the purpose of detecting metal. The security portals, or archway, will not harm the device, but it is prudent to walk through at a normal pace and not linger near them. However, the hand-held wand used by airport security personnel could deactivate some ICD devices if held directly over the pulse generator for a relatively short period of time. For this reason, ICD identification and security cards should be shown to airport security personnel, and patients are encouraged to request an alternative hand search. If security personnel insist on using the wand, the procedure should be performed quickly, and the wand should not linger over the device.

Patients with ICDs are also discouraged (or restricted) from professional automobile driving and are therefore not eligible for certain occupations, such as truck, bus or limousine driver, fireman, police officer, or pilot.

The reliability of implantable devices has come under scrutiny recently and it is important to understand the facts behind device reliability. ICDs *are* highly effective, but these are man-made devices, and flaws are bound to be identified and corrective action taken. A situation that attracted high public visibility in 2005, involved a number of recalled defibrillators from one manufacturer (Guidant). This situation was, in many ways, unique and particularly unfortunate. In this instance, the manufacturer did not disclose to physicians, patients, and the Food and Drug Administration (FDA) critical information regarding defective defibrillators that could short-circuit, fail, and result in death (initially, this occurred to a 21-year-old college student with HCM).

Now, the device manufacturers are working toward better ways to communicate such problems to physicians and patients. ICDs have saved thousands of lives and will save thousands more. Patients with HCM should not allow the events of 2005 to contaminate their trust in ICDs and those cardiologists who recommend and promote this life-saving therapy. To keep up to date on the reliability of your device, we recommend you maintain contact with the manufacturer of your device via their Internet sites or by telephone, and ask for the most recent information on your device at least once or twice per year. You can also talk to your electrophysiologist at the time of your ICD/pacemaker interrogation.

Support and advocacy groups

"Support groups" take a variety of forms, including the family unit and close friends. As individuals, however, we often find the need to discuss unique issues and problems, or find answers to complex questions that our family or friends may not be able to provide.

Such has been the substrate for creating support or advocacy groups focused on specific (often uncommon) medical conditions. Previously, such patient and disease-related support organizations were uncommon and located largely in local communities for the purpose of meeting directly to discuss common problems and sharing insights. This format allowed each person to seek the support of others affected by the same life circumstances they had experienced. More recently, the advent of the Internet has created an easier, inexpensive, and instantaneous free flow of information and contact between interested parties … in the context of on-line support groups, independent of geography or even international boundaries. This more efficient dissemination of information has made a substantial difference for patients with uncommon diseases such as HCM.

Most physicians understand the need for and benefits of support groups. Furthermore, many studies have shown that a positive attitude toward chronic disease has a direct influence on the patient's quality of life. Support groups offer patients and families the information and foundation with which to deal more effectively with their medical condition. In addition to a better quality of life for the patient, the entire family will benefit from a clearer understanding of the chronic disease (which in many cases is familial). The clarity achieved from the support group will also help patients communicate more effectively with physicians.

The Hypertrophic Cardiomyopathy Association (HCMA) was founded in 1996 by Lisa Salberg in the memory of her sister, Lori Anne Flanigan, who (although diagnosed years earlier) died suddenly of HCM. It was the aspiration of the founder to help others with HCM to have a complete, and unbiased understanding of their disease, as well as to provide a window (and access) to all available treatment options.

Indeed, one of the key elements of the HCMA is the facilitation of appropriate and accurate information by interfacing the patient (who is often confused about his/her disease) directly with the medical literature or clinicians expert in HCM. Frequently, patients with HCM are confused by the scientific literature – which can offer an exaggerated pessimism – or by a limited familiarity with HCM to which their own local cardiologist or internist may readily concede. However, the technological advance of the Internet has dramatically changed that state of affairs by substantially enhancing and embracing communication, and thereby offering HCM patients the opportunity to quickly become more appropriately informed regarding the nature and implications of their disease. In addition to the free flow of information via the Internet, the HCMA sponsors an annual national meeting in Morristown, New Jersey, which brings patients, families, clinical cardiologists, and researchers together to interact in a unique environment of partnership.

The specific goals and objectives of the HCMA are:

• To develop and maintain a network of support for people with HCM, their families, and the medical community

• To promote education about the symptoms, risks, and treatment options to those living with HCM, as well as access to expert professional care

• To raise awareness of protection against sudden death

• To develop and maintain a network of health care providers knowledgeable about the diagnosis and treatment of HCM

• To promote research in HCM, and provide ready access to this information

The HCMA provides a vast number of services to its membership including, but not limited to:

• Intimate, regionally located, person-to-person meetings

• Emotional support to individual patients and families with HCM

• Information about, and access to, medical providers

• Education to patients and the medical practitioners and community advocacy

• Internet-based access, including a message board

• International contacts to further the interest of its members

The HCMA also provides individual confidential support for matters related to:

• Concerns over a recent diagnosis

• Questions regarding "centers of excellence" in the field of HCM

• Information about all aspects of HCM and its treatment options

• Support to families who may have lost a relative or friend to HCM

• Access to other HCM patients with whom they share a unique bond

The HCMA provides those with HCM (or their family members) with the ability to make direct contact with other HCM patients. When you have been diagnosed with such a "rare" genetic disorder the access to others with the same problem provides a sense of belonging and the assurance that you are not alone.

Other international HCM Support Groups that you may contact:

In Canada:
HCMAC-Heart   www.HCMAC-Heart.ca
Suite 3138, 1010 Arbour Lake Rd NW
Calgary, Alberta, Canada, T3G 4Y8

In the United Kingdom:
The Cardiomyopathy Association
40 The Metro Centre, Tolpits Lane
Watford, Herts WD18SB U.K.

www.cardiomyopathy.org
Tel: +44 1923 249 977
Fax: +44 1923 249 987

In Australia and New Zealand:
Cardiomyopathy Association of
    Australia Ltd
P.O. Box 273
Hurstbridge, Victoria 3099, Australia

www.CMAA.org.au
Tel: +44 1300 552 622
Fax: +44 03 9499 1687

In Ireland:
Irish Heart Foundation
4 Clyde Road
Ballsbridge
Dublin 4, Ireland

www.irishheart.ie
Tel: +353 1 6685001
Fax: +353 1 6685896

In Israel:
The Israeli Hypertrophic Cardiomyopathy
    Association

gilead.org.il/ihcma/
Tel: +972 03 629 9389

In Italy:
Italian Hypertrophic Cardiomyopathy
    Institute
Via Jacopo Nardi 30
50132 Firenze, Italy

www.flownet.it/cmi/
Tel: +39 241 733
Fax: +39 241 027

In Germany:
The Heart.de
Stadtische Kliniken Bielefeld,
II. Medizinische Klinik,
TeutoburgerstraBe 50
33602 Bielefeld, Germany

www.theheart.de
Tel: +49 521 581 3431
Fax: +49 521 581 3499

For those who have had cardiac surgery:
The Mended Hearts, Inc.
7272 Greenville Avenue
Dallas, TX 75231-4596, USA

www.mendedhearts.org
Tel: +1 888 432 7899

What research is being conducted?

There are several active HCM research programs largely in the United States, Canada, Europe, and Japan. Research aimed at identifying and characterizing the genetic mutations and other abnormalities responsible for the disease are being performed in selected laboratories (in the United States, largely at Mayo Clinic and Brigham and Women's Hospital, Harvard Medical School). Other investigational efforts emphasize further definition and clarification of the diagnostic features and clinical course of HCM, as well as the development and application of novel treatment strategies. For example, introduction of the ICD for HCM has changed the course of the disease for many patients. However, as is true with many other relatively uncommon diseases, a limited number of clinical investigators are focusing their research interests on HCM. Consequently, financial support for HCM research is unfortunately sparse at present. Nevertheless, the ongoing research efforts in HCM are regarded as vigorous, although periodically changing in emphasis, but include clinical investigation focused on further definition of the disease spectrum, and determination of outcome and management strategies. Therefore, patients/physicians are encouraged to contact the HCMA for the most current information regarding HCM research and ways they can assist.

There are several centers with long-term commitments to clinical research in HCM. These include Minneapolis Heart Institute Foundation, Tufts-New England Medical Center, Mayo Clinic, Cleveland Clinic, St. Luke's Roosevelt Medical Center and Brigham and Woman's Hospital.

The 34 most frequently asked questions by patients about HCM, as addressed to the HCMA

1. *How did I get HCM?*

   HCM is a genetic disease. This means you were born with a mutation in a gene which causes HCM. You may not have had symptoms or known you had HCM, but nevertheless you were indeed born with the abnormal gene. However, what actually triggers the mutation itself to occur is unknown and environmental factors could conceivably play a role. Also, unknown is exactly how the mutation causes the heart (left ventricle) to thicken.

2. *I always have symptoms of dizziness, chest pain, and sometimes I am short of breath. I hesitate to bother my cardiologist, but when should I call him (her)?*

   You should discuss your symptom, in as much detail as appropriate, with your cardiologist. Ask what you should do if for any reason you feel you are in danger. You may be told to come to the office or go directly to an emergency room if your symptoms are more severe than usual.

3. *Should I have children?*

   This issue of genetic counseling does not lend itself easily to a "yes" or "no" answer, but is largely a matter of individual choice. It is a very common question from both the men and women members of the HCMA. HCM is an autosomal dominant disease, which means it is transmitted to about 50% of each consecutive generation. A child born to a parent with HCM has a statistical 50:50 chance of inheriting a mutant gene for HCM. However, it is important to remember that most people with HCM live normal lives without significant disability or the necessity of major medical interventions. Therefore, genetic counseling rarely advises against having children in absolute terms, although in those families with multiple sudden deaths or with other particularly serious disease manifestations, consideration should be given to not propagating what is obviously a malignant mutant gene.

   Women with HCM usually experience normal pregnancies, and there are no data suggesting that it is generally harmful to be pregnant with

HCM. In some cases a woman can remain on certain heart medications during the entire pregnancy (your obstetrician must be consulted on this point). Delivery may occasionally convey some added risks in selected patients with HCM. Epidural anesthesia has been associated with complications such as low blood pressure, and even a few reported deaths, and therefore we suggest that you discuss this strategy with your obstetrician well before delivery. If you choose to become pregnant you may also want to discuss breast feeding with your doctor to be sure your medications will not adversely affect the baby.

4. *Can I exercise? What types of daily recreational activities (or sports) can I participate in and what should I avoid?*

   Moderate exercise is fine, and patients with HCM are encouraged to be physically active. Walking, lap swimming, skating, golf, bowling, and yoga/tai-chi are examples of activities in which you may feel comfortable participating. You should consult with your cardiologist to tailor the most appropriate recreational exercise program to ensure that you are not placing yourself at undo and unnecessary risk.

   Particularly discouraged are those activities involving "burst" exertion in which the heart rate increases abruptly, such as sprinting, or any sports activity which create circumstances in which individuals cannot use their best judgment to stop and withdraw, given the onset of a sensation which could represent an HCM-related symptom. Finally, patients should avoid physical activities which provoke symptoms such as shortness of breath, chest pain, lightheadedness, or syncope. Helpful American Heart Association guidelines for recreational activities are presented in Table 1.

5. *Will HCM affect my sex life?*

   HCM, as well as some medications used to treat the disease, can cause fatigue so there may be a lack of energy rather than an absence of interest. However, medications used to treat HCM, such as beta-blockers, can occasionally cause impotence. In general, patients with HCM should be able to enjoy a normal sex life.

6. *I have thought about taking Viagra. Are there any risks specifically for HCM patients?*

   Probably. Due to its known pharmacologic actions (called peripheral vasodilation), it is assumed that Viagra could occasionally have adverse consequences (such as an increase in obstruction) in anyone with HCM, and probably should be avoided. The same rule applies to other drugs available to treat erectile dysfunction.

7. *Sometimes I think I am depressed. It is hard living with a chronic disease. What can I do to feel better?*

Do not be afraid to discuss your feelings with your physician. Depression can be a consequence of how you perceive your life situation, or possibly a side effect of a cardiac drug. Therefore, you may need to change medications to help relieve your depression. Whether or not a drug reaction is causing your depression, it might be prudent to see a psychiatrist, psychologist, or another mental health clinician to discuss your feelings. Certainly, living with a chronic disease *is* difficult and you should not hesitate to seek help in dealing with the emotional component of the condition. In families where there has been a death related to HCM, and other family members also have HCM, family/group counseling may prove helpful. Hopefully, some of the ideas in this book, and the HCMA website (www.4HCM.org), will also be useful.

8. *Will my heart get bigger?*

After reaching full maturity, normally by age 18–20 years, your heart growth usually stops. You may be made aware of slight changes in measurements of the thickness of the left ventricular wall, but generally the thickness will remain about the same. There are occasional exceptions, as in "adult-onset" hypertrophy. However, this rule covers an estimated 90–95% of the relevant clinical situations. You should not be concerned that your heart will grow perpetually – that is, increase in thickness throughout life, as there is always a point at which growth and thickening stop.

9. *I thought it was good to have big muscles, so what is wrong with a thick heart muscle?*

Having "big" muscles may sound like a good thing to some. However, an abnormally thick heart muscle is not beneficial to your health particularly if the thickening creates a situation in which the heart cannot properly fill with blood during the relaxation phase (diastole), or increases the risk for important arrhythmias when extreme … such as may occur in HCM.

10. *I live in a remote area, the local hospital is very small, and I am afraid they will not know how to help me. What can I do to help them help me?0*

Take a proactive role in your own health care. Stop by the local emergency room on a day you are feeling well and bring them information (such as this booklet). This will allow you the opportunity to speak to the staff when you are not in an emergency situation. By doing this you will provide those health care workers with the opportunity to understand HCM and your particular situation better, so that they will be ready for you in case you need them. The HCMA provides emergency information cards for patients to carry; please contact our office to obtain one. You may also request that the HCMA provide an information kit to your hospital or the physician's office. Simply e-mail the name and address of the health care provider to support@4HCM.org.

11. *I get very tired after a big meal, is this normal or is it my HCM?*

This is a very common complaint among HCM patients. There is, in fact, some evidence that a heavy meal can accentuate outflow obstruction in HCM and therefore symptoms such as shortness of breath. We suggest you eat smaller meals and try to avoid heavy foods. You will also want to avoid eating late at night.

12. *Are there any other conditions that cause HCM ... or can HCM cause any other conditions?*

There are syndromes that have been associated with a thick left ventricular wall closely resembling HCM. These include certain glycogen storage diseases which are metabolic conditions that resemble HCM clinically. Also, Noonan syndrome is associated with a thick heart muscle (but differs in its genetic basis from HCM). There are also other syndromes (some in infants) that may mimic HCM in appearance by virtue of a thick heart, but are not really the same disease. Danon disease and Pompe's disease are two such disorders, which differ distinctly from typical HCM by virtue of being metabolic glycogen storage diseases. HCM does not "cause" these other conditions.

13. *Is it usual to feel tired because of HCM?*

Yes, fatigue is probably the most common complaint we hear at the HCMA; however, it is a symptom which is distinctive from shortness of breath occurring with physical exertion. The basis for fatigue in HCM is not well understood.

14. *Can I drink caffeine? Eat salt?*

You should consult with your doctor for specific dietary restrictions and needs. Caffeine can have adverse reactions in some people and cause a racing heart. Therefore, if you are prone to arrhythmias you may want to avoid excessive caffeine products. Keep in mind that there are substantial amounts of caffeine in products other than coffee, such as Coca-Cola® (including Diet Coke®), tea, and chocolate. Excessive salt (sodium) may be harmful to those with high blood pressure or heart failure. In HCM, patients with low blood pressure, high sodium diets may be recommended. In contrast, if you are experiencing heart failure symptoms, sodium should be avoided. Your cardiologist can help you fully understand which situation fits your condition.

15. How important is my cholesterol level?

Just because you have HCM does not mean you are at any less risk for other forms of cardiovascular disease. Some older people with HCM also have high blood pressure and/or coronary artery disease due to atherosclerosis (mostly over age 50 years). Therefore, it is always a good idea to keep a "heart healthy" diet. On the other hand, HCM is not protective in any way against atherosclerosis.

16. Should I tell my cousins, aunts, uncles, or other blood relatives that I have been diagnosed with HCM?

Yes … because HCM is a genetic disease. Although it may be difficult to talk about this, you are obligated to let your family know. All blood relatives should be screened for HCM (with echocardiography, ECG, and consultation with a cardiologist); particularly if there have been premature deaths due to heart disease in the family.

17. Why can't they just cut my heart "down to size"?

That is not the answer to this disease. It would be medically untenable to remove enough abnormal muscle by surgery, or any other means, to "cure" a complex condition such as HCM. Even if that were possible, normalizing the heart structure would not necessarily solve the overall problem, since portions of the heart wall with normal thickness may also have abnormal function. Think of it this way … the real problem is at the cellular level. The removal of bulk still leaves improperly functioning cells which can impact negatively on your lifestyle. Of note, the myectomy operation does, by design, remove a portion of muscle from the ventricular septum. However, the surgeon only resects a small amount of tissue (i.e., 2–6 g); in hearts where the usual overall weight is about 500 g or more.

18. Can I drink alcohol?

There are little data on alcohol consumption in HCM, but moderation is advised. Alcohol can have a depressant effect on heart muscle function. Also, consumption of even a small amount of alcohol has been shown to increase the degree of obstruction, by acting as a stimulant. Drinking only in moderation is advised.

19. *What effect will marijuana have on someone with HCM?*

There is no direct evidence regarding this drug in patients with HCM. Nevertheless, it is the conservative (and prudent) position of the HCMA that marijuana should be avoided. Recent data in normal individuals shows that there is a 4-fold increase of myocardial infarction ("heart attack") after ingestion of marijuana. In addition, this drug increases the rate and the force of heart contractions. Marijuana could place a substantial burden on the HCM heart, especially with long-term use.

20. *What effect will the use of cocaine, heroin, or ecstasy or methamphet- amines have on someone with HCM?*

Although their precise actions with respect to HCM are not known with certainty, obviously, the use of these "recreational" drugs could prove to be adverse in someone with a complex disease such as HCM, and absolutely should be avoided. All of these drugs release metabolites which persistently increase heart rate and blood pressure. Cocaine itself can be responsible for sudden cardiac death due to inflammation of the heart muscle and weakening of the walls of the coronary arteries.

21. *Can I become a pilot?*

In the United States, a commercial pilot must pass a physical exami- nation annually for the FAA. At present, it is often possible to obtain a third-class (private aircraft) license with HCM. However, awarding a non-restricted first-class commercial license to a pilot with HCM is a controversial issue which may be associated with substantial admin- istrative difficulties.

22. *Are there any occupations I should avoid?*

You should probably avoid occupations that predominantly require particularly strenuous physical labor, prolonged driving, or positions responsible for public safety. In some HCM patients, intense physical activity undertaken chronically could prove detrimental, by conceiv- ably raising your risk for arrhythmias or sudden death. In addition, if you have an implanted device (pacemaker/defibrillator) you will need to avoid certain occupations such as those requiring contact with transmitting antennas and their power source, diathermy equipment (found in hospitals), power transmission lines, and electrical equip- ment (such as welders).

23. *Is a cure coming soon?*

You should not expect or anticipate HCM to be "cured." HCM is a complex, chronic disease, but one which can be managed or controlled in many ways. Major advances such as the implantable defibrillator may alter the natural history of the disease for many patients and restore an opportunity for normal or near-normal longevity. Although we have made great strides in identifying the genes that cause HCM, a cure (such as with gene therapy) may not be a reasonable aspiration due to the extremely complex and challenging scientific issues involved.

24. *Should I consult with an HCM specialist? How do you know if someone is an HCM specialist?*

The HCMA recommends that patients with HCM consult with a specialist in the field of HCM. Routine annual visits is the system that seems to work best in a chronic disease such as HCM, whether or not the patient perceives any clinical interval change. This may involve some travel because there are relatively few such cardiologists who have focused their professional energy on this disease. Although it is not always convenient to travel to an HCM specialist or center, in many cases such a strategy has made a substantial difference in the quality of care our HCMA members have received. It is also imperative to work with your hometown (local) cardiologist and keep the lines of communication open between all parties. An optimal situation is one in which your care involves both a knowledgeable local cardiologist and an HCM center (where you are routinely evaluated once a year).

The HCMA keeps a registry of all cardiologists who either have a special interest or experience with HCM, and are well respected by their peers.

25. *Can my child participate in competitive sports?*

Generally, no. Young patients with HCM are discouraged from participating in most intense competitive sports. There have been three national cardiology conferences (known as the Bethesda Conferences) over the last 20 years which have consistently made this recommendation. Exceptions to these exclusions are competitive golf and bowling (both with growing sports traditions in high school). This may be a very difficult adjustment for both parent and child. Of note, in the experience of the HCMA, there is no other clinical circumstance involving HCM in which there is the same capacity for emotion and misunderstanding as the recommendation to disqualify a young athlete from competitive sports because of HCM.

26. *Can my child participate in gym class?*

Participation in gym class will be dependent on your child's condition and the school system guidelines. If the child is capable of participating in basic activities the school doctor or nurse may work with the physical education teacher to tailor a realistic program. In some school systems this is called adaptive physical education. Therefore, you and the school should recognize that certain gym class sports activities may be intense and truly competitive in nature – for example, the traditional 600 yard run for time – and such physical activity should be avoided. It is most important to work these matters out prospectively and directly with the school … and in detail.

27. *Can I SCUBA dive?*

There is no information available that would suggest that the act of SCUBA diving itself creates physiologic alterations which are dangerous to HCM patients. However, SCUBA is usually a paired activity requiring submersion with a partner. Therefore, any impairment in consciousness, incapacitation, or onset of symptoms (due to HCM) would also unavoidably impact the safety of another person. For these reasons, this particular sporting activity is probably not advisable for patients with HCM.

28. *Why is HCM more common in men?*

Actually, it is not. HCM is an autosomal dominant genetic trait and, therefore, it occurs equally in men and women. However, it is obvious that HCM is recognized clinically much more commonly in men (about 60:40), suggesting that for a variety of reasons this disease is under-diagnosed in women.

29. *Are there additional problems that can occur from dehydration in HCM?*

Patients with HCM can have a significant increase in symptoms when dehydrated, often due to the occurrence or increase in obstruction and, therefore, should be very careful to maintain proper hydration by drinking adequate fluids on a daily basis.

30. *In the event of an emergency, should I or my family inform emergency service workers of my HCM diagnosis?*

Absolutely, you should inform them that you have HCM. You should also indicate that your ECG is abnormal as HCM patients sometimes have ECG patterns that can appear as if you have experienced a myocardial infarction ("heart attack") ... and you could be treated for a condition you do not have. Furthermore, you should inform the emergency personnel that nitroglycerine (a drug administered to "heart attack" victims) may aggravate chest pain/angina and other symptoms caused by HCM. Nitroglycerine is a vascular dilator and can cause severe hypotension (drop in your blood pressure) and promote obstruction, which could be dangerous to HCM patients.

31. Should I apply for disability if I have HCM?

No, not solely because you have HCM. However, you may want to consider this strategy if your symptoms limit your ability to function in the workplace. Disability is not granted based on diagnosis ... it is based on level of functional ability.

32. Isn't alcohol ablation an "easy" technique with little risk ... at least compared to surgery?

In reality, the risks of surgery in an experienced center are somewhat *less* than those for ablation, with no reported HCM-related operative deaths over the last decade at surgical centers such as Mayo Clinic, Cleveland Clinic, and Toronto General Hospital. Also, there is some concern that some young patients with alcohol ablation may have an increased risk for arrhythmias and sudden death over the long period of risk to which such individuals are exposed.

33. "Obstruction" sounds bad to me. Should I worry?

Obstruction to the flow of blood out of the left ventricle and into the aorta is a pressure gradient between the left ventricle and the aorta which raises pressure within the left ventricular chamber. It should be emphasized that this term does not at all imply total obstruction to flow, but only a partial obstruction caused by the mitral valve swinging forward to contact the ventricular septum during systole. Obstruction is very common in HCM ... 70% of patients have (or can generate) some obstruction ... which can cause progressive heart failure in certain patients, necessitating surgery.

34. What kind of health insurance should I have?

Any insurance coverage is better than no coverage at all. If at all possible Health Maintenance Organizations (HMOs) should be avoided in favor of Preferred Provider Organizations (PPO), Point of Service (without referral required) (POS), or indemnity plans. Many states offer plans for children at attractive rates and you should contact your local health department or school for more information on these programs. If you meet the financial requirements within your state, you may be eligible for a state or federally subsidized program, which may have many different names including Medicaid, State Children's Health Insurance Program (MD), Child Health Plus (NY), and Family Health Plus (NY). If you are on federal disability or are eligible for Social Security benefits based on age, you will likely qualify for Medicare health coverage. If you are on Medicare, it is advised that you also purchase a Medicare supplement.

Glossary

This is a list of scientific terms commonly used with regard to HCM, defined in a relatively straightforward fashion, but avoiding medical jargon, as much as possible. Some of these terms are also defined in the text, and are repeated here for completeness.

Ambulatory: Refers to tests performed when a person engages in their normal daily activities.

Aneurysm: A bulging outward of the left ventricular wall due to thinning and scarring in that area.

Angina: Chest pain, pressure, or discomfort usually brought on by exertion and relieved by rest. Angina results from insufficient oxygen supply to the heart muscle.

Angiography: An X-ray of the heart and blood vessels obtained at the time of cardiac catheterization with the injection of contrast dye. This test may be performed to assess the anatomy of the coronary arteries (blood vessels which supply the heart muscle).

Anticoagulation: Treatment to reduce the potential of blood to form clots (e.g., with heparin or warfarin). Such treatment is employed when there is a risk of clot formation in the heart, such as in the atria associated with atrial fibrillation.

Aorta: The main blood vessel which arises from the left ventricle and carries blood from the heart to the rest of the body.

Apex: The bottom portion of the heart; the tip of the left ventricle.

Arrhythmia: An abnormal rhythm or irregularity of the heartbeat. The heartbeat may either be too fast (*tachycardia*) or too slow (*bradycardia*). Arrhythmias may cause symptoms such as palpitation or lightheadedness or many have more serious consequences including sudden death.

Atria: The two filling chambers of the heart, one on the right and one on the left. Blood is collected in the atria while the ventricles are contracting. This blood is then released from the atria into the ventricles when they are ready to fill.

Atrial fibrillation: A common type of arrhythmia in which the atria lose their normal contraction pattern and the heart rhythm becomes irregular. Atrial fibrillation may be transient or persistent.

Cardiac arrest: When the heart ceases to have an effective rhythm and contraction, and death is imminent.

Cardiac catheterization: A special invasive test used in patients with many forms of heart disease, including selected patients with HCM. A fine tube (catheter) is passed from a blood vessel (in the arm or groin) into the heart, using X-ray guidance, and pressures within the heart chambers are measured. Heart structure and function can be assessed.

Cardiomyopathy: Refers to any disease predominantly involving the heart muscle; *cardia* refers to the heart and *myopathy* describes an abnormality of the heart muscle.

Concentric hypertrophy: The circumstance in which the left ventricular wall is thickened uniformly; also, referred to as symmetric hypertrophy. This is a rare pattern in HCM, which is usually asymmetric.

Congestive heart failure: A condition where weakness in the beating action of the heart causes fluid retention and symptoms of shortness of breath and fatigue on exercise. While this form of heart failure may occur in a few HCM patients with progressive disease, heart failure in HCM much more commonly occurs by a different mechanism related to the impaired relaxation and filling of the ventricles in diastole (and in the presence of normal beating action of the heart), or to obstruction.

Coronary artery disease: The common condition in which the coronary arteries (that deliver blood to the heart muscle) are narrowed by the accumulation of fatty plaque. When clots form on these plaques a "heart attack" (myocardial infarction) may result.

Diastole: Relaxation phase of the heart cycle when the ventricles passively fill with blood.

Diuretics: Drugs which increase the production of urine by the kidneys and decrease fluid retention.

Dominant inheritance: A disease which is transmitted to each consecutive generation, and occurs in about 50% of the relatives in a generation.

Echocardiogram: Commonly shortened to **echo**. Echocardiography is the single most important test in the assessment of HCM. This is a non-invasive ultrasound scan of the heart, which produces an image of the chambers, walls, and valves that can be viewed as a real-time movie (and is recorded permanently on videotape). *Doppler ultrasound* is part of the echocardiographic examination and produces a color-coded image of blood flow within the heart, detects areas of turbulent flow, and accurately measures the degree of obstruction. The pattern of filling of the left ventricle can also be assessed.

Electrocardiogram (or ECG): A very common test for all forms of heart disease. Electrodes are placed on the chest, wrists, and ankles to record electrical signals from the heart. Unlike the echocardiogram, the ECG does not produce a structural image of heart structure.

Electrophysiological study (or EPS): With this specialized test catheters are introduced into the heart during cardiac catheterization. These catheters can both record and stimulate the electrical activity of the heart. This test is rarely used in HCM now.

Endocarditis: An infection of the heart (usually of the valves) which can occur in HCM, although very rare. Bacteria in the bloodstream can adhere to the internal surface of the heart or abnormal heart structures, particularly the mitral valve in HCM.

Exercise stress testing: Exercise capacity may be tested using either a treadmill or a stationary bicycle. During an exercise test, a physician and technician monitor the patient's performance as well as symptoms, ECG, and blood pressure; sometimes the consumption of oxygen is also measured. When combined with an echocardiogram, the possibility of obstruction occurring with exercise can be assessed.

Genes and chromosomes: Genes are the code or blueprint which build all the tissues in the body. Each individual has thousands of genes and they are all present in every cell of the body. Genes come in pairs, one inherited from the mother and the other from the father. In each cell the genes are grouped together by tiny, thread-like structures called chromosomes. Each person has 23 pairs of chromosomes.

HCMA: The Hypertrophic Cardiomyopathy Association, a patient support and advocacy organization. More information is available at www.4HCM.org.

Heart attack: Not the appropriate terminology to describe a sudden collapse in HCM, but rather is common terminology for an acute myocardial infarction due to atherosclerosis and coronary artery disease.

Heart block: Occasionally the normal electrical signal cannot travel into the ventricles due to a pathologic disruption in the conducting system;

a slow heart rate results. This situation can be identified by an ECG and corrected with a pacemaker.

HOCM: Acronym for "hypertrophic obstructive cardiomyopathy" which is still commonly used in the United Kingdom. However, this term implies that the disease is *always* characterized by stenosis and outflow obstruction which, of course, is not the case.

Holter monitor: A continuous ambulatory recording of the heartbeat over 24–48 hours. Adhesive electrodes are placed on the chest, with wires that connect to a special cassette recorder which is worn on a belt. A Holter monitor detects irregularity of the heartbeat, otherwise known as arrhythmia.

Hypertrophy: Literally means an increase in the muscle mass (or weight) of the heart. In HCM, hypertrophy refers specifically to an excessive thickening of the left ventricular wall.

IHSS: Acronym for "idiopathic hypertrophic subaortic stenosis" which is an older name for HCM, used primarily in the United States in the 1960s. Of course, this term implies that the disease is always characterized by stenosis (i.e., outflow obstruction), which is erroneous.

Implantable cardioverter-defibrillator (ICD): A specialized and sophisticated device which is permanently implanted. It senses when the heart rate is excessively fast (which may represent a potentially lethal arrhythmia) and responds by either delivering a low-energy electrical shock or pacing the heart to restore the normal heart rhythm. ICDs can also serve as a pacemaker to pace the heart when the heart rate is too slow. Nevertheless, the ICD should not be confused with the conventional pacemaker. These are very different instruments with different objectives … although all ICDs do *also* contain pacemaker function.

Mitral regurgitation: Refers to blood leaking back through the mitral valve during ejection. This occurs in HCM when there is outflow tract obstruction, but may vary considerably in degree.

Murmur: A murmur is caused by turbulent blood flow within the heart. In HCM the characteristic murmur is due to outflow obstruction and the turbulence produced by systolic anterior motion of the mitral valve, or the associated mitral regurgitation. Not all murmurs, however, are of significance in patients with HCM and your doctor may regard your murmur as "innocent" and unrelated to the disease.

Mutation: A genetic defect that causes a permanent change in the normal DNA code.

Myectomy (or myotomy-myectomy): An operation which may be performed in severely symptomatic patients with HCM to remove a portion of the thickened muscle from the upper portion of the ventricular septum, and thereby relieve the outflow tract obstruction. This procedure is usually associated with long-lasting improvement of symptoms.

Myocardial disarray: When heart tissue from patients with HCM is viewed under a microscope the normal parallel alignment of the muscle cells (myocytes) is usually absent. Instead, characteristic of HCM, these cells (or bundles of cells) appear disorganized ... or in disarray ... that is arranged at perpendicular and oblique angles to each other. There is no clinical test that can specifically detect disarray.

Myocardium: The specialized muscle tissue which makes up the walls of the heart. It is this part of the heart which is most abnormal in HCM.

Myosin: A protein within muscle cells which is prominently involved in normal contraction. Often in HCM, the gene that is responsible for coding myosin is abnormal and accounts for the disease in some families.

Non-invasive: Refers to tests that generally do not invade the integrity of the body, such as echocardiography or electrocardiography. Cardiac catheterization, in which catheters are introduced through blood vessels into the heart, is an example of an invasive test.

Outflow obstruction: Produced by the contact between mitral valve and thickened ventricular septum during the ejection phase of the heart cycle. This results in a pressure *gradient* between the upper and lower portions of the left ventricular cavity ... and high pressures within the left ventricular chamber. Therefore, the terms *gradient* and *obstruction* are used synonymously.

Outflow tract: The short channel in the heart through which blood ultimately passes from the left ventricle into the aorta. It is essentially the upper portion of the left ventricle.

Pacemaker: When the normal electrical impulse fails to be transmitted to the ventricles a pacemaker can be implanted to correct this problem. This involves inserting a small box containing a battery under the skin in the chest area, connected to fine wires, which are inserted into a vein and then into the heart, in order to deliver the necessary impulses.

Palpitation: An uncomfortable awareness of the heartbeat or rhythm. Palpitations may be due to normal heartbeats made more prominent by anxiety or exercise, or may in fact be caused by an arrhythmia. The presence of palpitations *per se* does not necessarily convey any prognostic significance in HCM, although on occasion (particularly when prolonged) they may be important signs about which you should advise your doctor.

Septum (ventricular septum): That portion of the heart wall which divides the cavities of the right and left ventricles. In HCM, muscle thickening is usually most marked and most common in the septum. This observation has led to the descriptive term, asymmetric septal hypertrophy.

Systole: The phase of heart cycle when blood is forcibly ejected from the ventricles – that is, blood in the left ventricle flows into the aorta and to the major arteries and organs of the body.

Systolic anterior motion of the mitral valve (or SAM): In some patients with HCM, the mitral valve moves forward and touches the septum (there should normally be a considerable gap between these two structures) during the ejection of blood from the heart, thereby partially blocking the flow of blood from the left ventricle into the aorta. In the vast majority of patients, SAM is the mechanism of obstruction in HCM.

Ventricles: The two main (lower) pumping chambers of the heart, the right and left ventricle pump blood to the lungs and aorta, respectively. The left ventricle is that portion of the heart most commonly and predominantly affected in HCM.

Ventricular tachycardia: A potentially serious arrhythmia in which repetitive and rapid premature beats arise within the ventricles, and can lead to lethal ventricular fibrillation.

Key HCM references

Arad M, Maron BJ, Gorham JM, Johnson WH Jr., Saul JP, Perez-Atayde AR, Spirito P, Wright GB, Kanter RJ, Seidman CE, Seidman JG. Glycogen storage diseases presenting as hypertrophic cardiomyopathy. N Engl J Med 2005;352:362–72.

Elliot PM, Gimeno JR, Thaman R, Shah J, Ward D, Dickie S, Tome MT, McKenna WJ. Historical trends in reported survival rates in patients with hypertrophy cardiomyopathy. Heart 2006;92:785–91.

Fibroozi S, Elliott PM, Sharma S, et al. Septal myotomy-myectomy and transcoronary septal alcohol ablation in hypertrophic obstructive cardiomyopathy. A comparison of clinical, hemodynamic, and exercise outcomes. Eur Heart J 2002;23:1617–1624.

Hauser RG, Maron BJ. Lessons from the failure and recall of an implantable cardioverter defibrillator. Circulation 2005;112:2040–2042.

Kimmelstiel CD, Maron BJ. Role of percutaneous septal ablation in hypertrophic obstructive cardiomyopathy. Circulation 2004;109:452–456.

Kitaoka H, Doi Y, Casey SA, Hitomi N, Furuno T, Maron BJ. Comparison of prevalence of apical hypertrophic cardiomyopathy in Japan and the United States. Am J Cardiol 2003;92:1183–1186.

Maron BJ. Hypertrophic cardiomyopathy: A systematic review. J Am Med Assoc 2002;287:1308–1320.

Maron BJ. Sudden death in young athletes. N Engl J Med 2003;349:1064–1075.

Maron BJ. Hypertrophic cardiomyopathy: An important global disease (Editorial). Am J Med 2004;116:63–65.

Maron BJ. Surgery for hypertrophic obstructive cardiomyopathy: Alive and quite well. Circulation 2005;111:2016–2018.

Maron BJ, Zipes DP. 36th Bethesda Conference: Eligibility Recommendations for Competitive Athletes with Cardiovascular Abnormalities. J Am Coll Cardiol 2005;45: 1312–1375.

Maron BJ, Thompson PD, Puffer JC, McGrew CA, Strong WB, Douglas PS, Clark LT, Mitten MJ, Crawford MH, Atkins DL, Driscoll DJ, Epstein AE. Cardiovascular preparticipation screening of competitive athletes. Circulation 1996;94:850–856.

Maron BJ, Casey SA, Poliac LC, Gohman TE, Almquist AK, Aeppli DM. Clinical course of hypertrophic cardiomyopathy in a regional United States cohort. J Am Med Assoc 1999;281:650–655.

Maron BJ, Nishimura RA, McKenna WJ, Rakowski H, Josephson ME, Kieval RS. Assessment of permanent dual-chamber pacing as a treatment for drug-refractory symptomatic patients with obstructive hypertrophic cardiomyopathy: A randomized, double-blind cross-over study (M-PATHY). Circulation 1999;99:2927–2933.

Maron BJ, Olivotto I, Spirito P, Casey SA, Bellone P, Gohman TE, Graham KJ, Burton DA, Cecchi F. Epidemiology of hypertrophic cardiomyopathy-related death: Revisited in a large non-referral based patient population. Circulation 2000;102:858–864.

Maron BJ, Shen W-K, Link MS, Epstein AE, Almquist AK, Daubert JP, Bardy GH, Favale S, Rea RF, Boriani G, Estes NAM III, Spirito P, Casey SA, Stanton MS, Betocchi S.

Efficacy of implantable cardioverter-defibrillators for the prevention of sudden death in patients with hypertrophic cardiomyopathy. N Engl J Med 2000;342: 365–373.

Maron BJ, Casey SA, Hauser RG, Aeppli DM. Clinical course of hypertrophic cardiomyopathy with survival to advanced ages. J Am Coll Cardiol 2003;42:882–888.

Maron BJ, Estes NAM III, Maron MS, Almquist AK, Link MS, Udelson J. Primary prevention of sudden death as a novel treatment strategy in hypertrophic cardiomyopathy. Circulation 2003;107:2872–2875.

Maron BJ, Barry JA, Poole RS. Pilots, hypertrophic cardiomyopathy and issues of aviation and public safety. Am J Cardiol 2004;93:441–444.

Maron BJ, Chaitman B, Ackerman MJ, Bayés de Luna A, Corrado D, Crosson JE, Deal BJ, Driscoll DJ, Estes NAM III, Araújo CG, Liang DH, Mitten MJ, Myerburg RJ, Pelliccia A, Thompson PD, Towbin JA, Van Camp SP. American Heart Association Scientific Statement: Recommendations for Physical Activity and Recreational Sports Participation for Young Patients with Genetic Cardiovascular Diseases. Circulation 2004;109:2807–2816.

Maron BJ, Dearani JA, Ommen SR, Maron MS, Schaff HV, Gersh BJ, Nishimura RA. The case for surgery in obstructive hypertrophic cardiomyopathy. J Am Coll Cardiol 2004;44:2044–2053.

Maron BJ, McKenna WJ, Danielson GK, Kappenberger LJ, Kuhn HJ, Seidman CE, Shah PM, Spencer WH, Spirito P, ten Cate FJ, Wigle ED. Pocket Guidelines on Hypertrophic Cardiomyopathy. Joint Task Force on Clinical Expert Consensus Documents of the American College of Cardiology Foundation and the European Society of Cardiology Committee for Practice Guidelines, 2004, pp. 1–16.

Maron MS, Zenovich AG, Casey SA, Link MS, Udelson JE, Aeppli DM, Maron BJ. Significance and relation between magnitude of left ventricular hypertrophy and heart failure systems in hypertrophic cardiomyopathy. Am J Cardiol 2005;95: 1329–1333.

Matthews T, Dickinson J. Considerations for delivery in pregnancies complicated by maternal hypertrophic obstructive cardiomyopathy. Aust N Z J Obstet Gynaecol 2005;45:526–528.

McCully RB, Nishimura RA, Tajik AJ, Schaff HZ, Danielson GK. Extent of clinical improvement after surgical treatment of hypertrophic obstructive cardiomyopathy. Circulation 1996;94:467–471.

Nishimura RA, Holmes DR. Hypertrophic obstructive cardiomyopathy. N Engl J Med 2004;350:1320–1327.

Nishimura RA, Trusty JM, Hayes DL, Ilstrup DM, Larson DR, Hayes SN, Allison TG, Tajik AJ. Dual-chamber pacing for hypertrophic cardiomyopathy: A randomized, double-blind cross-over study. J Am Coll Cardiol 1997;29:435–441.

Olivotto I, Cecchi F, Casey SA, Dolara A, Traverse JH, Maron BJ. Impact of atrial fibrillation on the clinical course of hypertrophic cardiomyopathy. Circulation 2001;104: 2517–2524.

Ommen SR, Maron BJ, Olivotto I, Maron MS, Cecchi F, Betocchi S, Gersh BJ, Ackerman MJ, McCully RB, Dearani JA, Schaff HV, Danielson GK, Tajik AJ, Nishimura RA. Long-term effects of surgical septal myectomy on survival in patients with obstructive hypertrophic cardiomyopathy. J Am Coll Cardiol 2005;46:470–476.

Qin JX, Shiota T, Lever HM, et al. Outcome of patients with hypertrophic obstructive cardiomyopathy after percutaneous transluminal septal myocardial ablation and septal myectomy surgery. J Am Coll Cardiol 2001;38:1994–2000.

Rickers C, Wilke NM, Jerosch-Herold M, Casey SA, Panse P, Panse N, Weil J, Zenovich AG, Maron BJ. Utility of cardiac magnetic resonance imaging in the diagnosis of hypertrophic cardiomyopathy. Circulation 2005;112:855–861.

Seggewiss H, Gleichman U, Faber L, et al. Percutaneous transluminal septal myocardial ablation in hypertrophic obstructive cardiomyopathy: Acute results and 3-month follow-up in 25 patients. J Am Coll Cardiol 1998;31:252–258.

Sherrid MV, Barac I, McKenna WJ, Elliott PM, Dickie S, Chojnowska L, Casey S, Maron BJ. Multicenter study of the efficacy and safety of disopyramide in obstructive hypertrophic cardiomyopathy. J Am Coll Cardiol 2005;45:1251–1258.

Spirito P, Rapezzi C, Bellone P, et al. Infective endocarditis in hypertrophic cardiomyopathy. Prevalence, incidence and indications for antibiotic prophylaxis. Circulation 1999;99:2132–2137.

Spirito P, Bellone P, Harris KM, Bernabo P, Bruzzi P, Maron BJ. Magnitude of left ventricular hypertrophy predicts the risk of sudden death in hypertrophic cardiomyopathy. N Engl J Med 2000;342:1778–1785.

Van Driest SL, Ommen SR, Tajik AJ, Gersh BJ, Ackerman MJ. Yield of genetic testing in hypertrophic cardiomyopathy. Mayo Clin Proc 2005;80:739–744.

van Langen IM, Birnie E, Schuurman E, Tan HL, Hofman N, Bonsel GJ, Wilde AA. Preferences of cardiologists and clinical geneticists for the future organization of genetic care in hypertrophic cardiomyopathy: A survey. Clin Genet 2005;68:360–368.

Woo A, Williams WG, Choi R, Wigle ED, Rozenblyum E, Fedwick K, Siu S, Ralph-Edwards A, Rakowski H. Clinical and echocardiographic determinants of long-term survival after surgical myectomy in obstructive hypertrophic cardiomyopathy. Circulation 2005;111:2033–2041.

Yang Z, McMahon CJ, Smith LR, Bersola J, Adesina AM, Breinholt JP, Kearney DL, Dreyer WJ, Denfield SW, Price JF, Grenier M, Kertesz NJ, Clunie SK, Fernbach SD, Southern JF, Berger S, Towbin JA, Bowles KR, Bowles NE. Danon disease as an underrecognized cause of hypertrophic cardiomyopathy in children. Circulation 2005;112:1612–1617.

Appendix

Guidelines for Commercial Genetic Testing: Laboratory for Molecular Medicine. *Harvard Medical School – Partners Healthcare Center for Genetics and Genomics.* www.hpcgg.org/LMM.

Hypertrophic cardiomyopathy genetic test

Background

Hypertrophic cardiomyopathy (HCM) is a primary disorder of the myocardium that is characterized by unexplained left ventricular hypertrophy (LVH) in a non-dilated ventricle. Distinctive findings of myocardial hypertrophy with myocyte disarray are the histopathologic hallmarks of this disorder. The clinical spectrum of HCM is diverse, ranging from asymptomatic individuals to those with disabling symptoms of heart failure, exercise intolerance, and chest pain. HCM is also associated with an increased risk of sudden cardiac death.

Genetic studies have defined HCM as a disease of the sarcomere (see Figure A-1) – caused by mutations in any of 11 genes that encode different elements of the contractile apparatus in cardiac myocytes. To date, about 400 individual mutations have been identified. With a prevalence estimated to be approximately 1/500 to 1/1000 in the general population, HCM is the most common monogenic cardiac disorder and is inherited in an autosomal dominant mode.

Echocardiographic evidence of unexplained left ventricular hypertrophy typically forms the basis for establishing the clinical diagnosis of HCM; however, this finding fails to identify all affected individuals. Although the gene mutations responsible for causing HCM are inherited at the time of conception, it may take decades before there is a clinically evident expression of LVH. Therefore, making the clinical diagnosis of HCM early in life may be a particular challenge.

In addition to confirming the diagnosis of HCM in patients with clinically evident disease, genetic testing allows for early identification and diagnosis of individuals at greatest risk for developing HCM, prior to the expression of typical clinical manifestations (e.g., LVH). If a mutation is identified in such a preclinical individual, regular and serial outpatient follow-up is indicated. Referral to a cardiologist with specific expertise in the management of HCM is highly recommended for patients with established disease as well as family members who are found to be genotype positive. Longitudinal

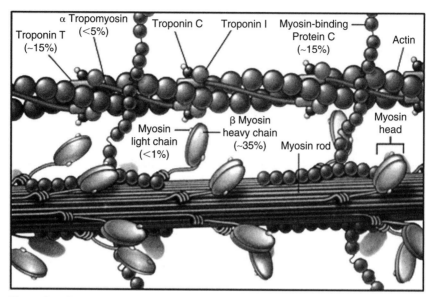

Figure A-1 Some of the sarcomere genes responsible for HCM.

study is necessary to survey for the development of clinical manifestations as well as to optimize treatment. If clinically unaffected members of a family with an identified causal mutation for HCM are found not to carry that mutation (genotype negative), they can be definitively diagnosed as unaffected with HCM and reassured that neither they nor their offspring will be at higher risk compared to the general population to develop this disorder. The need for serial follow-up is also obviated.

Genetic testing for HCM is performed by screening for mutations via direct DNA sequencing of the coding regions of the genes most commonly implicated in causing HCM. The test is offered in two panels: panel A (HCM-A) includes the five most common genes for HCM: *MYH7*, *MYBPC3*, *TNNT2*, *TNNI3*, and *TPM1*. The overall detection rate of a pathogenic mutation for HCM-A among patients with clinically evident HCM is approximately 50–60%. Panel B (HCM-B) includes three additional genes, *ACTC*, *MYL2*, and *MYL3*, and the detection rate of a pathogenic mutation for HCM-B is approximately 5–10%, making the combined detection rate 55–70% if both panels are tested.

Synonyms (OMIM#192600)
- VENTRICULAR HYPERTROPHY, HEREDITARY
- ASYMMETRIC SEPTAL HYPERTROPHY; ASH

- HYPERTROPHIC SUBAORTIC STENOSIS, IDIOPATHIC; IHSS
- CARDIOMYOPATHY, FAMILIAL HYPERTROPHIC; FHC

HCM genetic tests
- Direct DNA sequencing will be performed to detect mutations in the genes most commonly associated with HCM.

HCM-A

Gene	Name	OMIM#	Locus
MYH7	Myosin, heavy chain 7	160760	14q12
MYBPC3	Myosin-binding protein C, cardiac	600958	11p11.2
TNNT2	Troponin-T2, cardiac	191045	1q32
TNNI3	Troponin-I, cardiac	191044	19q13.4
TPM1	Tropomyosin 1	191010	15q22.1

HCM-B

Gene	Name	OMIM#	Locus
ACTC	Actin, alpha, cardiac muscle	102540	15q14
MYL2	Myosin regulatory light chain	160781	12q23-q24.3
MYL3	Myosin essential light chain, cardiac	160790	3p

Epidemiology: 1/500 to 1/1000
- Males and females are affected in equal frequency
- No known racial predilection.

Clinical features (variable, and may not occur in every patient):
- Left ventricular hypertrophy (LVH)
- Electrocardiograph (EKG) changes
- Shortness of breath, chest pain, exercise intolerance
- Increased risk of sudden cardiac death (SCD)

Inheritance pattern: Autosomal dominant
- The presence of a pathogenic mutation in one copy of the above listed genes is sufficient to cause HCM.
- Children of an affected individual with an identified pathogenic mutation have a 50% risk of inheriting the same mutation.

Test indications
- Patients with clinical features of HCM.
- Parents, siblings, and possibly children of a patient diagnosed with a mutation in one of the HCM genes.

Test outcomes
- The detection of a pathogenic mutation will offer a definitive diagnosis for an affected patient.
- Referral to a cardiology center with expertise in the management of HCM is highly recommended.

Turn-around-time:
- Turn-around-time: 6 weeks

Methodology
Bi-directional sequence analysis is performed on 106 exons and splice sites in five genes in HCM-A, or on 19 exons and splice sites in three genes in HCM-B. These tests do not detect additional mutations in non-coding regions that could affect gene expression or deletions encompassing a large portion of the gene.

Test accuracy
This assay has greater than 99.9% accuracy to detect mutations in the sequence analyzed.

Test sensitivity
The overall detection rate of mutations by screening patients with clinical symptoms of HCM is:

Panel	Detection rate (%)
HCM-A	50–60
HCM-B	5–10
Both	55–70

Cost and CPT codes
Mutation screening of five genes by sequencing: HCM-A
- Cost: $3000.00
- CPT codes: 83891(1), 83894(1), 83898(94), 83904(94), 83912(1)

Mutation screening of additional three genes by sequencing: HCM-B
- Cost: $1150.00
- CPT codes: 83891(1), 83894(1), 83898(19), 83904(19), 83912(1)

Sequencing for the family members of patients with an identified mutation
- Cost: $250.00
- CPT codes: 83891(1), 83894(1), 83898(1), 83904(1), 83912(1)

Recently, panel C (cost $1,500) has been added for glycogen storage cardiomyopathies which mimic sarcomeric HCM—LAMP 2 and PRKAGZ.

Specimen collection and shipping guidelines

Specimen requirements

For diagnostic, presymptomatic and carrier testing:
- 7 ml of whole blood (3–5 ml for an infant) in a lavender top tube (K_aEDTA)
- 10 µg of DNA in a 1–2 ml screw top tube. Please provide DNA concentration
- Send in sample with completed requisition form and have patient sign consent on back of form: www.hpcgg.org/LMM/regform

A saliva sample is acceptable for the following tests:
- Known mutation testing for all gene tests currently offered
- *PTPN11* gene test
- In place of the blood sample required *EGFR* testing (see *EGFR* sample requirements)

Please contact the Laboratory for Molecular Medicine (LMM) to have a saliva collection kit mailed to you.

Shipping

The Laboratory accepts samples Monday to Friday from 9 a.m. to 5 p.m. Samples should be sent overnight at room temperature and accompanied by a completed requisition form with a signed consent. Please ship samples to:

Laboratory for Molecular Medicine
Attention: Clinical Laboratory
65 Landsdowne Street
Cambridge, MA 02139

Please follow specific regulations set depending on courier service utilized.

Hypertrophic Cardiomyopathy Association
Membership Application

If you would like to become a member of the association which will entitle you to receive copies of regular newsletters, benefit from a local contact network, and access advice and counseling please complete and return this form.

If you do not wish to join but feel that you can help us by making a contribution please send your donation to the address below.

Please check the appropriate box.

❏ I would like to become a member of the association and enclose $50.00 to cover the annual subscription renewable annually September 1.

❏ Please check this box if you do not wish your name and telephone number to be given to other members.

❏ I enclose a donation to the Hypertrophic Cardiomyopathy Association for the amount of _____. I would like to direct my donation to:
  ❏ General Operation
  ❏ Research Fund
  ❏ Scholarships

Checks should be made payable to HCMA and returned with this form to:

HCMA
P.O. Box 306
328 Green Pond Rd.
Hibernia, NJ 07842
Attn: Membership

Tel: 973-983-7429 or
Toll free: 877-329-4262
Fax: 973-983-7870
E-mail: support@4hcm.org

DR/MR/MRS/MISS (Circle as appropriate)

Last name _____ First name _____

Address _____

City/State _____ Zip Code _____

Home Phone _____ Work Phone _____

E-mail _____ Date of birth _____

Date of Diagnosis _____ Present Date _____

Index

Note: Italicized page numbers refer to figures and tables.

DISCARD

DATE DUE

ILL 4/30/10	

DEMCO INC. 38-2931